Sleep Science Made Simple

Alen Juginović

Sleep Science Made Simple

A Clear and Concise Guide

Springer

Alen Juginović
Department of Neurobiology
Harvard Medical School
Boston, MA, USA

ISBN 978-3-031-92062-2 ISBN 978-3-031-92060-8 (eBook)
https://doi.org/10.1007/978-3-031-92060-8

This Springer imprint is published by the registered company Springer Nature Switzerland AG
The registered company address is: Gewerbestrasse 11, 6330 Cham, Switzerland

Foreword

Sleep remains one of the most fascinating and complex aspects of human biology. As a physician and researcher at Harvard Medical School (Rogulja Lab) studying the impact of sleep quality on health, I've witnessed firsthand how proper sleep can transform lives—and how its absence can devastate them. This book emerges from years of experience and research, driven by a simple observation: despite spending roughly a third of our lives asleep, most of us know remarkably little about this crucial biological process. For example, some of the most basic questions like "Why do we sleep 7-9 hours and not 2 or 4 hours" remain unanswered.

I regularly encounter people struggling with sleep issues that affect their health, work, and relationships. Many come with misconceptions about sleep, often having tried various remedies without understanding the underlying biology of their sleep problems. Others dismiss sleep as a luxury rather than the biological necessity it truly is. This growing disconnects between our understanding of sleep and its fundamental importance to our health has become a critical public health challenge.

This book aims to bridge that knowledge gap. Rather than offering quick fixes or one-size-fits-all solutions, it presents the latest scientific understanding of sleep in an accessible way. You'll learn how your brain regulates sleep, why different sleep stages matter, and how sleep affects everything from your immune system to your mental health. Importantly, you'll learn about the most common sleep disorders and understand how this knowledge translates into practical strategies for improving sleep.

The science of sleep has advanced dramatically in recent years. We now know that sleep isn't simply a period of rest—it's an active process essential for physical repair, memory consolidation, emotional regulation, and immune function. Through advanced imaging techniques and molecular research, we're uncovering new aspects of sleep's role in health and disease. This book synthesizes these discoveries into a comprehensive, yet easily understandable exploration of sleep biology that will help you understand and even optimize sleep.

Whether you're a healthcare professional seeking to better understand your patients' sleep issues, someone struggling with sleep problems, or simply curious about the science of sleep, this book offers valuable insights into one of our most essential biological processes. My hope is that by understanding sleep better, you'll not only improve your own rest but also appreciate why sleep deserves priority in our increasingly fast-paced world. After all, sleep isn't time wasted—it's an investment that you make today for a healthier tomorrow.

Department of Neurobiology
Harvard Medical School
Boston, MA, USA

Alen Juginović

Special Thanks

If You Want to Go Fast, Go Alone. If You Want to Go Far, Go Together.

This African proverb has shaped my perspective throughout my journey. Since my earliest days in kindergarten and continuing through elementary school, high school, and medical school, these words have served as a constant principle in my approach to life.

I will never forget the amazing people who have helped shape me into the person I am today. I wouldn't have graduated from the School of Medicine in Split, Croatia, if it weren't for my dedicated teachers and professors who constantly motivated me to work harder from elementary school to medical school. A turning point in my student life was when I became a student assistant at the Department of Neuroscience. I am grateful for the team at the Neuroscience Department and the Center for Sleep Medicine in Split, Croatia, St. Catherine Specialty Hospital (Zagreb, Croatia), as well as the Rogulja Lab (and prof. Dragana Rogulja) at Harvard Medical School (Boston, MA, USA) who have made such a positive impact on my life. I wouldn't be where I am today if it weren't for the incredible colleagues, students, professors, and staff who have taught me so much about life. I am also grateful for the friends who have supported me through tough times and celebrated my successes with me. A big thanks goes to my family, grandparents, cousins, and broader family members who have always believed in me and my abilities. And lastly, I am grateful to my parents, Gordana and Davor, who have always been there for me.

Even though some of these amazing people are no longer with us, I will always be thankful for the impact they have had on my life. In life, you must never put limitations on yourself and always believe that anything is possible. Stay grounded, be a good person, be thankful for the opportunities you receive, and never forget your true friends and family who are always there for you. Always remember that good things will eventually come back to you. Dream big and live life to the fullest!

Disclaimer

The information provided in this book is based on current scientific research and is intended for educational purposes only. It should not be used as a substitute for professional medical advice, diagnosis, or treatment. While the author has made every effort to ensure the accuracy and completeness of the information contained in this book, some details may become outdated as new research emerges.

If you suspect you have a sleep disorder or other medical condition, please consult with a qualified healthcare provider. The author and publisher are not responsible for any adverse effects or consequences resulting from the use of any suggestions, preparations, or procedures described in this book.

References to specific research findings, statistics, and medical studies were current at the time of publication (2024/2025). The field of sleep science continues to evolve, and readers are encouraged to consult recent scientific literature and healthcare providers for the most up-to-date information.

Contents

Part I The Science of Sleep

1 The Brain Behind Sleep 3
1.1 Your Brain: The Sleep Command Center 3
References 7

2 Understanding the Essence of Sleep 9
2.1 The Nature of Sleep: How and Why We Sleep 9
References 13

3 The Circadian Rhythm 15
3.1 The Circadian Clock: Our Body's Internal Timekeeper 15
3.1.1 How Light Controls the Brain's Internal Clock 19
3.1.2 Modern Life Versus Your Circadian Clock 21
References 24

4 Sleep Labs: How We Study Sleep 27
4.1 The Tools We Use to Study Sleep 27
4.1.1 Consumer Sleep Tech: Innovations and Current Challenges 29
References 30

5 Inside the Sleeping Brain: From Chemistry to Dreams 33
5.1 Brain at Night: Molecular and Electrical Foundations of Sleep and Its Stages 33
5.1.1 The Molecular Mechanisms Behind Our Brain's Transition from Wake to Sleep 33
5.1.2 The Temperature-Sleep Connection: How Body Temperature Affects Our Rest 36
5.1.3 Understanding the Stages of Sleep 38
5.1.4 Dreams and Brain Activity 45
5.1.5 Sleep Versus Anesthesia: Two Different Paths to Altered Consciousness 46
References 47

6 Nutrition and Sleep: Dietary Influences on Rest . . . 51
6.1 Food, Drinks, and Sleep: How Diet Affects Our Rest . . . 51
6.1.1 Caffeine and the Sleep-Wake Cycle . . . 51
6.1.2 What We Eat Affects How We Sleep . . . 53
6.1.3 Alcohol and Sleep: A Deceptive Relationship . . . 54
6.1.4 Sleep Supplements: What Works and What Doesn't . . . 55
References . . . 56

Part II Sleep: A Foundation of Health and Longevity

7 Sleep as a Key Pillar for Health Optimization . . . 61
7.1 Beyond Rest: Sleep's Critical Role in Health Optimization . . . 61
References . . . 62

8 Sleep and Cognitive Performance: Learning, Memory, and Mental Clarity . . . 65
8.1 Sleep's Role in Learning and Cognitive Effects of Poor Sleep . . . 65
References . . . 69

9 Sleep's Role in Mental Health . . . 71
9.1 Sleep and Mental Health: A Two-Way Street . . . 71
9.1.1 Sleep and Depression . . . 73
9.1.2 Sleep and Anxiety . . . 74
9.1.3 Sleep and Bipolar Disorder . . . 75
9.1.4 Sleep and Schizophrenia . . . 75
References . . . 76

10 Stress, Sleep, and the Body's Adaptive Response . . . 79
10.1 Sleep and Stress: A Vicious Cycle . . . 79
References . . . 82

11 Immunity and Rest . . . 83
11.1 Sleep and Immune Function: A Critical Partnership . . . 83
References . . . 84

12 Sleep's Influence on Your Metabolism . . . 87
12.1 Sleep's Impact on Metabolic Health . . . 87
References . . . 88

13 The Role of Sleep in Cardiovascular Health . . . 89
13.1 Sleep and Cardiovascular Health . . . 89
References . . . 90

14 How Sleep Supports Brain Health . . . 91
14.1 Sleep and Brain Health . . . 91
References . . . 93

15 When Work Disrupts Sleep: Occupational Health Consequences . . . 95
15.1 Sleep, Shift Work, and Cancer . . . 95
References . . . 96

16 Balancing Between Too Little and Too Much Sleep ... 99
16.1 Balancing Sleep: The Risk of Sleep Deprivation and Oversleeping ... 99
References ... 100

17 Sleep's Role in Productivity, Leadership, and Economic Outcomes ... 101
17.1 Sleep in the Business World ... 101
17.1.1 The High Price of Poor Sleep: Implications for Leadership and the Economy ... 101
17.1.2 From Fatigue to Focus: How Modern Workplaces Can Prioritize Sleep Health ... 103
References ... 105

18 The Crucial Role of Sleep for Athletes ... 107
18.1 Sleep and Athletes ... 107
References ... 110

Part III The World of Sleep Disorders

19 The World of Sleep Disorders ... 113
19.1 Understanding Sleep Disorders: A Modern Health Challenge ... 113
References ... 114

20 Customizing Sleep Treatments: A Targeted Approach to Health ... 117
20.1 Personalizing Sleep Treatment: Beyond One-Size-Fits-All ... 117
Reference ... 118

21 Insomnia ... 119
21.1 Insomnia—The Most Prevalent Sleep Disorder ... 119
21.1.1 Understanding Insomnia: The Search for Sleep ... 119
21.1.2 Diagnosing and Treating Insomnia ... 121
References ... 124

22 Sleep Apnea ... 125
22.1 Sleep Apnea—When Breathing Stops ... 125
22.1.1 Sleep Apnea: An Introduction ... 125
22.1.2 Understanding Sleep Apnea's Reach: Risk Factors and Prevalence ... 126
22.1.3 Different Types of Sleep Apnea ... 127
22.1.4 Diagnosing and Treating Sleep Apnea ... 130
22.1.5 The Long-Term Impact of Untreated Sleep Apnea ... 133
References ... 135

23 Restless Leg Syndrome and Periodic Limb Movement Disorder ... 137
23.1 When Legs Won't Rest: Restless Legs Syndrome and Periodic Limb Movement Disorder ... 137
23.1.1 What Are Restless Legs Syndrome and Periodic Limb Movement Disorder? ... 137
23.1.2 Treatment Options ... 138
References ... 139

24 Circadian Rhythm Disorders 141
24.1 Circadian Rhythm Disorders: When Your Body's Clock Is Disrupted 141
24.1.1 Introduction 141
24.1.2 Diagnostic and Treatment Approaches: Resetting the Biological Clock 142
References 144

25 Parasomnias 145
25.1 Parasomnias: When Sleep Gets Strange 145
25.1.1 Introduction to Parasomnias 145
25.1.2 Non-REM Parasomnias 146
25.1.3 REM Parasomnias 146
25.1.4 Other Sleep-Related Behaviors 146
25.1.5 Diagnosing and Treating Parasomnias 147
References 148

26 Better Sleep at Home 149
26.1 Optimizing Your Sleep at Home 149

27 Future of Sleep Science 153
27.1 Looking Forward: The Future of Sleep Science and Medicine 153

Index 155

About the Author

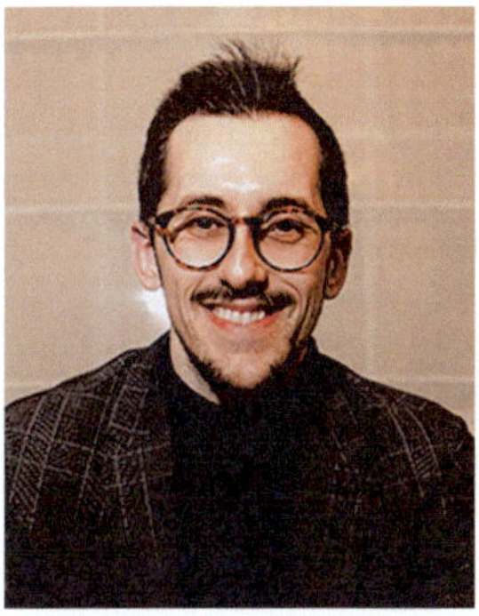

Alen Juginović is a physician and postdoctoral researcher at Harvard Medical School's Department of Neurobiology (Rogulja Lab) in Boston, MA, USA, studying how poor sleep affects health. He teaches "Neurobiology of Emotions and Mood Disorders" at Harvard College and serves on the Editorial Board of the *Journal of Clinical Sleep Medicine*, the official journal of the American Academy of Sleep Medicine. As a sleep consultant, he works with elite athletes and teams, business professionals, and frequent travelers to optimize their sleep patterns and manage jet lag. He also advises and invests in several sleep technology startups.

During his medical studies at the University of Split School of Medicine in Croatia, Alen demonstrated exceptional leadership. He founded the Society for Neuroscience, served as Student Council president, and organized international conferences that brought Nobel Laureates to Croatia. After graduating in 2018, he continued building initiatives that bridge international biomedical communities. He co-founded Med&X, a Croatian NGO that accelerates Croatian biomedical development through three key programs:

– **Plexus Conference** and similar conferences organized by the same Med&X team, which have welcomed over 2500 participants, 10 Nobel Laureates, and numerous global biomedical leaders from more than 30 countries since 2017

– **Med&X Accelerator**, collaborating with research labs and clinics from leading institutions like Mayo Clinic, Cleveland Clinic, Mass General Brigham, Harvard University, and Yale University to provide internship opportunities for Croatian medical professionals and students

– **Med&X Biomedical Forum**, which is a leading platform that unites Croatian and international leaders in medicine, science, and business to foster collaboration,strategic initiatives and advancement of Croatian biomedicine

As President of the Boston Chapter of the Association of Croatian American Professionals, Alen strengthens ties within the Croatian community in Greater Boston. He frequently delivers keynote speeches at international biomedical conferences and is a reviewer for several scientific journals. His contributions have earned recognition including the 2024 Rising Star by the Association of Croatian American Professionals, 2021 European Citizen's Prize, Think Global Award 2020 in the Community category, and Best Young Project Manager in Croatia 2020. He was also shortlisted for Forbes "30 under 30" in Healthcare and Science in Europe.

For scientific collaboration, speaking opportunities, or other inquiries, contact Alen at juginovic.alen@gmail.com.

List of Figures

Part I

Fig. 1 Transitional 0. (Image generated using the prompt "Soft dandelion; close up; warm colour illustration," by Adobe, Adobe Firefly, 2024. (https://firefly.adobe.com/)) 1

Fig. 1.1 Structure and organization of the human brain and neuron ("Created in BioRender. Juginovic, A. (2025) https://BioRender.com/q40d911") 4

Fig. 1.2 Illustration showing the organisation of the central and peripheral nervous systems ("Image generated by ChatGPT (OpenAI), 2025. Used with permission") 6

Fig. 2.1 How your sleep changes with age. ("Stacked area analysis was performed using GraphPad Prism version 10.4.1. for Windows, GraphPad Software, www.graphpad.com") 10

Fig. 2.2 The human sleep cycle pattern. ("Image generated by ChatGPT (OpenAI), 2025. Used with permission") 11

Fig. 3.1 Neural circuit of sleep-wake regulation. ("Created in BioRender. Juginovic, A. (2025) https://BioRender.com/u57d964") 16

Fig. 3.2 Simplified molecular regulation of the circadian rhythm. ("Created in BioRender. Juginovic, A. (2025) https://BioRender.com/f03n895") 17

Fig. 3.3 Anatomical organization of the hypothalamus. ("Created in BioRender. Juginovic, A. (2025) https://BioRender.com/t75q493") 20

Fig. 3.4 Illustration of the body's biological clock across a 24-h day. ("Image generated by ChatGPT (OpenAI), 2025. Used with permission") 21

Fig. 4.1 Standard sleep study equipment (Polysomnography). ("Created in BioRender. Juginovic, A. (2025) https://BioRender.com/b30w055") 28

Fig. 4.2 Sleep stage distribution through the night. ("Created in BioRender. Juginovic, A. (2025) https://BioRender.com/k07m798") 29

Fig. 5.1 Key brain regions involved in sleep regulation. ("Created in BioRender. Juginovic, A. (2025) https://BioRender.com/y91d094"). 34
Fig. 5.2 Body temperature during sleep. ("Created in BioRender. Juginovic, A. (2025) https://BioRender.com/n99v409") 36
Fig. 5.3 Types of brain wave activity. (''Created in BioRender. Juginovic, A. (2025) https://BioRender.com/q69f078") 38
Fig. 5.4 Schematic overview of characteristics of N1 sleep stage. ("Image generated by ChatGPT (OpenAI), 2025. Used with permission"). 40
Fig. 5.5 Schematic overview of characteristics of N2 sleep stage. ("Image generated by ChatGPT (OpenAI), 2025. Used with permission") 41
Fig. 5.6 Schematic overview of characteristics of N3 sleep stage. ("Image generated by ChatGPT (OpenAI), 2025. Used with permission") 42
Fig. 5.7 Schematic overview of characteristics of REM sleep stage. ("Image generated by ChatGPT (OpenAI), 2025. Used with permission") 44

Fig. 6.1 Visual guide to Tryptophan-rich foods and melatonin-rich foods. ("Image generated by ChatGPT (OpenAI), 2025. Used with permission") 54

Part II
Fig. 1 Transitional 1. (Image generated using the prompt "White bed and pillows; modern style illustration," by Adobe, Adobe Firefly, 2024. (https://firefly.adobe.com/)) 59

Fig. 10.1 The hypothalamic-pituitary-adrenal (HPA) axis: stress response mechanism. ("Created in BioRender. Juginovic, A. (2025) https://BioRender.com/t71h717") 80

Fig. 14.1 The glymphatic system: brain waste clearance pathway. ("Created in BioRender. Juginovic, A. (2025) https://BioRender.com/r33y434") 92

Fig. 17.1 Schematic overview of the hidden cost of poor sleep—how sleep deprivation impacts the economy. ("Image generated by ChatGPT (OpenAI), 2025. Used with permission") 103

Fig. 18.1 Illustrative overview of how poor sleep undermines athletic performance and injury recovery. ("Image generated by ChatGPT (OpenAI), 2025. Used with permission") 108

Part III
Fig. 1 Transitional 2. (Image generated using the prompt "Soft sunset clouds in sky; modern style illustration," by Adobe, Adobe Firefly, 2024. (https://firefly.adobe.com/)) 111

Fig. 21.1 Illustration showing the key symptoms of insomnia. ("Image generated by ChatGPT (OpenAI), 2025. Used with permission") 121

Fig. 22.1 Obstructive sleep apnea (**a**—Physiological state, **b**—Obstructive sleep apnea). ("Created in BioRender. Juginovic, A. (2025) https://BioRender.com/i01r459") 126

Fig. 22.2 CPAP therapy: continuous airflow support for sleep apnea treatment. ("Image generated by ChatGPT (OpenAI), 2025. Used with permission") 131

Fig. 26.1 Wide-ranging health impacts of poor sleep. ("Created in BioRender. Juginovic, A. (2025) https://BioRender.com/x14v509") 151

Part I

The Science of Sleep

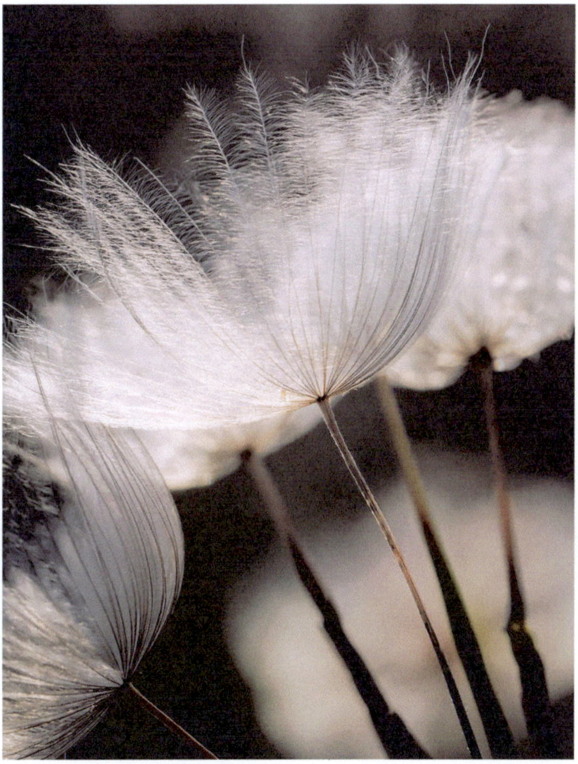

Fig. 1 Transitional 0. (Image generated using the prompt "Soft dandelion; close up; warm colour illustration," by Adobe, Adobe Firefly, 2024. (https://firefly.adobe.com/))

The Brain Behind Sleep

1

1.1 Your Brain: The Sleep Command Center

Have you ever wondered why some people can fall asleep instantly while others lie awake for hours? Or why your morning alarm feels like torture some days but not others? The answers lie in an extraordinary organ and possibly the most complex thing we are trying to understand—the brain. Every night, as you drift off to sleep, so many processes unfold in your brain that affect everything from your mood to your ability to fight off a common cold. While sleep might seem simple—just close your eyes and drift off—the biology behind it reveals that sleep may well be one of the body's most sophisticated biological processes.

Before we make the complex world of sleep and biological rhythms simple for you, let's understand the basic parts and functions of your brain that make sleep possible. Think of your brain as the control center of your body—a remarkably complex organ that weighs about one and a half kilograms (three pounds) and contains roughly 70–90 billion nerve cells (neurons) alongside 40–130 billion support cells called glia [1, 2]. These glial cells, once thought to be mere "brain glue," actually play crucial roles in supporting and protecting neurons, helping them communicate, and maintaining brain health [3]. The brain never truly shuts down, even during sleep. Instead, it remains active 24 h a day, processing information, controlling bodily functions, and maintaining the delicate balance between sleep and wakefulness. Every morning when you wake up feeling refreshed, it's because your brain has been hard at work throughout the night, overseeing various restoration processes.

The brain consists of several key regions, each playing specific roles in sleep and wakefulness. At its base is the brainstem, which connects your brain to your spinal cord. The brainstem contains centers that control basic functions like breathing and heart rate, and it plays a vital role in regulating sleep and wakefulness [4]. When you're sleeping peacefully, your brainstem ensures that you keep breathing steadily and your heart continues beating regularly, even though you're completely unaware of these processes. Above the brainstem sits the hypothalamus, about the size of an almond, which houses important sleep-control centers, including your master

A. Juginovic, *Sleep Science Made Simple*,
https://doi.org/10.1007/978-3-031-92060-8_1

circadian clock in a small part called the suprachiasmatic nucleus (SCN) [5]. This tiny region called the SCN, containing only about 20,000 neurons, acts as your body's primary timekeeper, coordinating daily rhythms of sleep and wake, hormone release, and temperature regulation with the external environment [6].

Neurons form the foundation of all brain activity. Neurons are remarkable cells, distinct from most others in your body due to their specialized ability to form vast communication networks (Fig. 1.1). These brain cells can rapidly exchange information with each other and, most importantly, create new connections based on your experiences. When you learn something new—whether it's riding a bike or memorizing a phone number—your neurons form and strengthen connections with each other. This amazing ability of your brain to rewire itself is called neuroplasticity, and it continues throughout your entire life, even during sleep when your brain processes and consolidates the day's experiences [7]. Neurons communicate using both electrical and chemical signals in a process that occurs billions of times every second. When a neuron becomes activated, it generates a tiny electrical impulse called an action potential that travels along its length at speeds up to around 450 miles per hour [8]. This incredible speed explains how you can react almost instantly to stimuli, whether it's catching a falling object or responding to your alarm clock in the morning. When this electrical signal reaches the end of the part of the neuron called the axon, it triggers the release of chemical messengers called neurotransmitters. These chemicals cross small gaps between neurons, passing messages to neighboring cells by attaching to specific receptors. This process

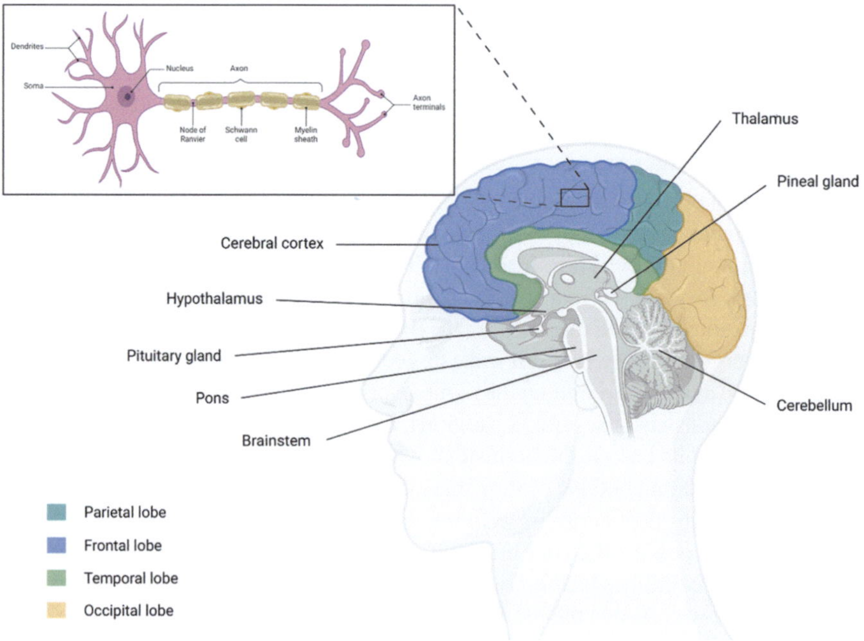

Fig. 1.1 Structure and organization of the human brain and neuron ("Created in BioRender. Juginovic, A. (2025) https://BioRender.com/q40d911")

happens countless times every second throughout your brain, creating complex patterns of activity that control everything from your thoughts and emotions to your sleep patterns. Think of neurotransmitters as the brain's text messages, sending specific instructions that determine, e.g., whether you feel alert or sleepy.

Several key neurotransmitters control sleep and wakefulness, working like a complex system of switches. While these neurotransmitters perform many different functions throughout the brain and body, they play particularly important roles in regulating sleep. GABA (gamma-aminobutyric acid) acts as your brain's main "off switch," reducing the activity of other neurons and promoting sleep. GABA fulfills this role by inhibiting or slowing down the activity of neurons—imagine it as a natural brake pedal that helps your brain shift into a quieter, calmer state that promotes sleep [9]. When GABA levels rise in the evening, you begin to feel that familiar sense of drowsiness. Another important sleep promoter is adenosine, which gradually builds up in your brain throughout the day, increasing what we call "sleep pressure"[10]. The longer you stay awake, the more adenosine accumulates, making you feel increasingly sleepy. In contrast, neurotransmitters like norepinephrine and acetylcholine act as "on switches," promoting wakefulness and alertness (although they also play roles in modulating certain sleep stages) [11, 12]. Your brain carefully balances these chemical signals throughout the day and night, which explains why you feel energetic at certain times and sleepy at others. This delicate chemical balance also explains why substances that affect these neurotransmitters, such as caffeine (which blocks adenosine receptors) or certain medications, (e.g. antidepressants) can significantly impact your sleep patterns [13].

Hormones—chemical messengers that travel through your bloodstream—play crucial roles in sleep regulation. Unlike neurotransmitters that work locally in the brain, hormones can affect cells throughout your entire body. Melatonin, often called the "sleep hormone," is produced by the pineal gland (a small pea-sized gland deep in your brain) and increases in the evening to help prepare your body for sleep [14]. While your brain's master circadian clock (in the suprachiasmatic nucleus) controls melatonin production, this hormone serves a crucial role in synchronizing the daily rhythms of cells in your entire body [15]. Nearly every cell in your body contains its own molecular clock—these are called peripheral clocks—and melatonin helps keep them all operating in harmony with the master clock and with each other [16]. These cellular timekeepers help each tissue optimize its function according to the time of day, ensuring that processes like metabolism, hormone production, and cell repair happen at the right times. For example, your liver needs to know when you're likely to eat, and your muscles need to prepare for daily activity. Your brain typically starts producing melatonin about 2–3 h before your natural bedtime, which explains why you gradually become sleepy as the evening progresses [17]. Cortisol, known as the "stress hormone", typically peaks in the early morning hours, helping you wake up and start your day [18]. This explains why many people naturally feel most alert in the morning, even without caffeine. Other hormones also follow daily rhythms—growth hormone reaches its highest levels during deep sleep, while thyroid stimulating hormone (TSH) peaks in the evening [19, 20]. These hormones work together to maintain your daily sleep-wake rhythm.

Your nervous system extends far beyond your brain, forming an extensive communication network throughout your body (Fig. 1.2). The central nervous system consists of your brain and spinal cord, acting like the main processing unit and primary "cable" of a computer. The peripheral nervous system includes all the nerves throughout your body, similar to a complex network of wires carrying information to and from every part of your body. This network at least partly explains why sleep affects your entire body—from your muscles and organs to your immune system. When you feel physically tired, mentally exhausted, or both, it's because this network is signaling your brain that rest is needed.

Within the peripheral nervous system, the autonomic nervous system controls your body's automatic functions and operates in two complementary modes, each essential for proper sleep. The sympathetic nervous system—your "fight or flight" response—increases e.g. heart rate and alertness [21]. This system may be too active if you're having a hard time falling asleep, like when you're stressed or excited. The parasympathetic nervous system, nicknamed the "rest and digest" system, does the opposite—slowing your heart rate and promoting relaxation [21]. When you're lying in bed feeling peaceful and drowsy, that's your parasympathetic system at work. These systems alternate dominance throughout the day, with the parasympathetic system taking control as bedtime approaches. Your brain contains

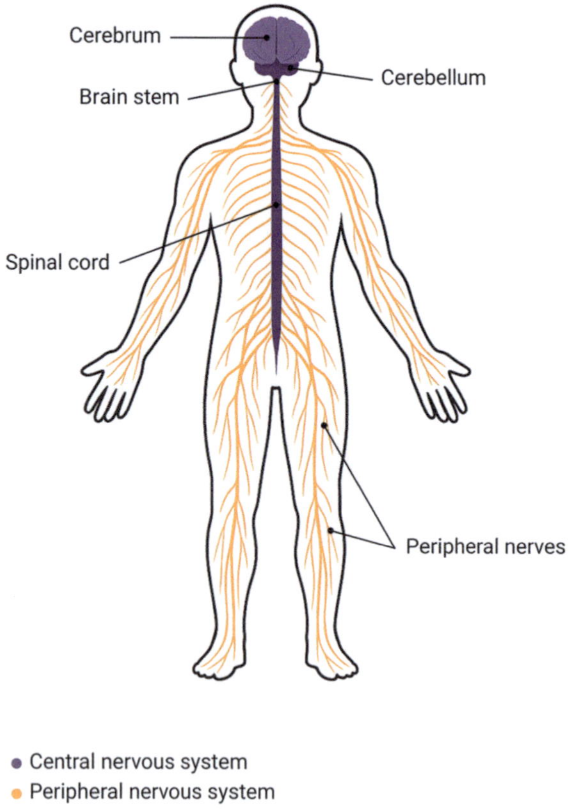

Fig. 1.2 Illustration showing the organisation of the central and peripheral nervous systems ("Image generated by ChatGPT (OpenAI), 2025. Used with permission")

specialized circuits dedicated to sleep and wakefulness, forming what scientists call the sleep-wake system. This system works like a complex switch, determining when you feel sleepy or alert. One key component is the ascending reticular activating system (ARAS), a network of neurons in your brainstem that acts like your brain's "power switch" [22]. This system helps maintain wakefulness and can quickly shift you from sleep to alertness when needed—like when a loud noise wakes you up or when your alarm goes off in the morning. It receives input from your senses and helps determine whether you should stay asleep or wake up based on environmental cues. We'll explore these and other wake and sleep circuits in more detail in a later chapter.

Temperature regulation, closely tied to sleep, involves the hypothalamus working as your body's thermostat [23]. Your core body temperature naturally fluctuates throughout the day, dropping by about 1 °C (2 °F) during sleep [24]. This temperature drop actually helps initiate and maintain sleep, which might explain why it's easier to fall asleep in a cool room than a warm one. Your brain coordinates this temperature rhythm with other sleep-related processes, creating optimal conditions for rest and recovery.

This system of brain regions, neurons, neurotransmitters, and hormones creates the foundation for healthy sleep. When you understand these basics, many common sleep experiences begin to make sense. That overwhelming drowsiness you feel late in the evening? It's the result of rising melatonin levels and accumulating sleep pressure from adenosine buildup. The natural awakening in the morning? That's your biological clock activating wake-promoting circuits and triggering the release of cortisol. Your difficulty sleeping when stressed? That's your sympathetic nervous system remaining active when your parasympathetic system should be taking over. Of course all of these are simplified explanations, and as we explore sleep throughout this book, we'll learn more details about the "sleep system" and see how it can sometimes go wrong, and equally importantly, what you can do to help it work at its best.

References

1. Goriely A. Eighty-six billion and counting: do we know the number of neurons in the human brain? Brain. 202427:awae390. PMID: 39602822.
2. von Bartheld CS, Bahney J, Herculano-Houzel S. The search for true numbers of neurons and glial cells in the human brain: a review of 150 years of cell counting. J Comp Neurol. 2016;524(18):3865–95. PMID: 27187682.
3. Jäkel S, Dimou L. Glial cells and their function in the adult brain: a journey through the history of their ablation. Front Cell Neurosci. 2017;11:24. PMID: 28243193.
4. Benarroch EE. Brainstem integration of arousal, sleep, cardiovascular, and respiratory control. Neurology. 2018;91(21):958–66. PMID: 30355703.
5. Szymusiak R, Gvilia I, McGinty D. Hypothalamic control of sleep. Sleep Med. 2007;8(4):291–301. PMID: 17468047.
6. Ramkisoensing A, Meijer JH. Synchronization of biological clock neurons by light and peripheral feedback systems promotes circadian rhythms and health. Front Neurol. 2015;6:128. PMID: 26097465.

7. Innocenti GM. Defining neuroplasticity. Handb Clin Neurol. 2022;184:3–18. PMID: 35034744.
8. DeMaegd ML, Städele C, Stein W. Axonal conduction velocity measurement. Bio Protoc. 2017;7(5):e2152. PMID: 34458468.
9. Ganguly K, Schinder AF, Wong ST, Poo M. GABA itself promotes the developmental switch of neuronal GABAergic responses from excitation to inhibition. Cell. 2001;105(4):521–32. PMID: 11371348.
10. Jagannath A, Varga N, Dallmann R, Rando G, Gosselin P, Ebrahimjee F, Taylor L, Mosneagu D, Stefaniak J, Walsh S, Palumaa T, Di Pretoro S, Sanghani H, Wakaf Z, Churchill GC, Galione A, Peirson SN, Boison D, Brown SA, Foster RG, Vasudevan SR. Adenosine integrates light and sleep signalling for the regulation of circadian timing in mice. Nat Commun. 2021;12(1):2113. PMID: 33837202.
11. Becchetti A, Amadeo A. Why we forget our dreams: acetylcholine and norepinephrine in wakefulness and REM sleep. Behav Brain Sci. 2016;39:e202. PMID: 28347366.
12. España RA, Scammell TE. Sleep neurobiology from a clinical perspective. Sleep. 2011;34(7):845–58. PMID: 21731134.
13. Reichert CF, Deboer T, Landolt HP. Adenosine, caffeine, and sleep-wake regulation: state of the science and perspectives. J Sleep Res. 2022;31(4):e13597. https://doi.org/10.1111/jsr.13597. PMID: 35575450.
14. Masters A, Pandi-Perumal SR, Seixas A, Girardin JL, McFarlane SI. Melatonin, the hormone of darkness: from sleep promotion to ebola treatment. Brain Disord Ther. 2014;4(1):1000151. PMID: 25705578.
15. Pfeffer M, Korf HW, Wicht H. Synchronizing effects of melatonin on diurnal and circadian rhythms. Gen Comp Endocrinol. 2018;258:215–21. PMID: 28533170.
16. Smith JG, Sassone-Corsi P. Clock-in, clock-out: circadian timekeeping between tissues. Biochem (Lond). 2020;42(2):6–10. PMID: 34083887.
17. Doghramji K. Melatonin and its receptors: a new class of sleep-promoting agents. J Clin Sleep Med. 2007;3(5 Suppl):S17–23. PMID: 17824497.
18. Mohd Azmi NAS, Juliana N, Azmani S, Mohd Effendy N, Abu IF, Mohd Fahmi Teng NI, Das S. Cortisol on circadian rhythm and its effect on cardiovascular system. Int J Environ Res Public Health. 2021;18(2):676. PMID: 33466883.
19. Vakili H, Jin Y, Cattini PA. Evidence for a circadian effect on the reduction of human growth hormone gene expression in response to excess caloric intake. J Biol Chem. 2016;291(26):13823–33. PMID: 27151213.
20. Persani L, Terzolo M, Asteria C, Orlandi F, Angeli A, Beck-Peccoz P. Circadian variations of thyrotropin bioactivity in normal subjects and patients with primary hypothyroidism. J Clin Endocrinol Metab. 1995;80(9):2722–8. PMID: 7673415.
21. Murtazina A, Adameyko I. The peripheral nervous system. Development. 2023;150(9):dev201164. PMID: 37170957.
22. Jones BE. Neurobiology of waking and sleeping. Handb Clin Neurol. 2011;98:131–49. PMID: 21056184.
23. Zhao ZD, Yang WZ, Gao C, Fu X, Zhang W, Zhou Q, Chen W, Ni X, Lin JK, Yang J, Xu XH, Shen WL. A hypothalamic circuit that controls body temperature. Proc Natl Acad Sci USA. 2017;114(8):2042–7. PMID: 28053227.
24. Szymusiak R. Body temperature and sleep. Handb Clin Neurol. 2018;156:341–51. PMID: 30454599.

Understanding the Essence of Sleep

2

2.1 The Nature of Sleep: How and Why We Sleep

Sleep is a whole-body process, driven by a network of brain regions, neurons, neurotransmitters, and hormones that together lay the foundation for healthy rest. When you understand these basics, many common sleep experiences begin to make sense. That overwhelming drowsiness you feel late in the evening? It's the result of rising melatonin levels and accumulating sleep pressure from adenosine buildup. The natural awakening in the morning? That's your biological clock activating wake-promoting circuits and triggering the release of cortisol. Your difficulty sleeping when stressed? That's your sympathetic nervous system remaining active when your parasympathetic system should be taking over.

When we sleep, specific regions of our brain become highly active, sometimes even more active than during wakefulness [1]. Using advanced brain imaging techniques like functional magnetic resonance imaging (fMRI) which measures blood flow, scientists can observe activity in different brain regions. These studies have revealed surprising patterns: while some areas of the brain reduce their activity during sleep, others spring into action. The hippocampus, a region crucial for memory formation, shows particularly intense activity during specific sleep stages, suggesting a vital role in processing the day's experiences, particularly memory [2]. Meanwhile, the prefrontal cortex, responsible for complex decision-making, enters a period of relative quiet, potentially explaining why our judgment becomes impaired when we're sleep-deprived [3].

Sleep is composed of four different sleep stages, N1 (light sleep), N2, N3 (slow wave or deep sleep) and REM (Rapid Eye Movement) sleep, each serving specific functions. a typical night, your body progresses through these stages in a complete sleep cycle lasting approximately 90–110 min, repeating this cycle 4–5 times throughout the typical night. During sleep, three main changes occur: our senses become less responsive to the outside world, our voluntary muscles become still, and our brain operates in a distinct mode that differs significantly from wakefulness [4]. These changes aren't just incidental—they help create the ideal conditions for

A. Juginović, *Sleep Science Made Simple*,
https://doi.org/10.1007/978-3-031-92060-8_2

the brain to perform its restorative functions. Think of these changes as your brain's "night shift" preparations. Just as a building needs quiet hours for maintenance and cleaning, your brain requires specific conditions to carry out its nighttime duties. While asleep, your brain performs several critical functions. It converts short-term memories into long-term storage while simultaneously repairing tissues, growing muscle, and releasing growth hormone [5–7]. Your immune system gets a boost as your body produces essential immune components [7]. The brain processes the day's emotional experiences and regulates mood, while also balancing hormones that control appetite and energy use [8]. Perhaps most remarkably, sleep allows your brain to clear out metabolic waste products that accumulate during wakefulness through a specialized cleaning system called the glymphatic system, which works like your brain's nighttime cleanup crew [9]. The brain accomplishes the aforementioned functions through different sleep stages. In deeper sleep stages (stage N3), physical restoration and hormone release take priority, while REM (Rapid Eye Movement) sleep focuses on emotional processing and memory consolidation—all while keeping muscles paralyzed to ensure safety during dreams, which most frequently occur in REM sleep [10]. After all, you don't want to physically act out your dreams during REM sleep, right?

The amount of sleep we need changes throughout our lives, reflecting the different demands placed on our bodies and brains at various life stages (Fig. 2.1). Adults between 18 and 65 years need 7–9 h of sleep each night, but the exact amount varies among individuals within this range [11]. Newborns require up to 18 h of sleep daily, even though their sleep is not consolidated in a single nightly bout [11, 12]. One of the misconceptions is that older people need less sleep, but the fact is that they still need a minimum of 7 h which many unfortunately cannot get due to

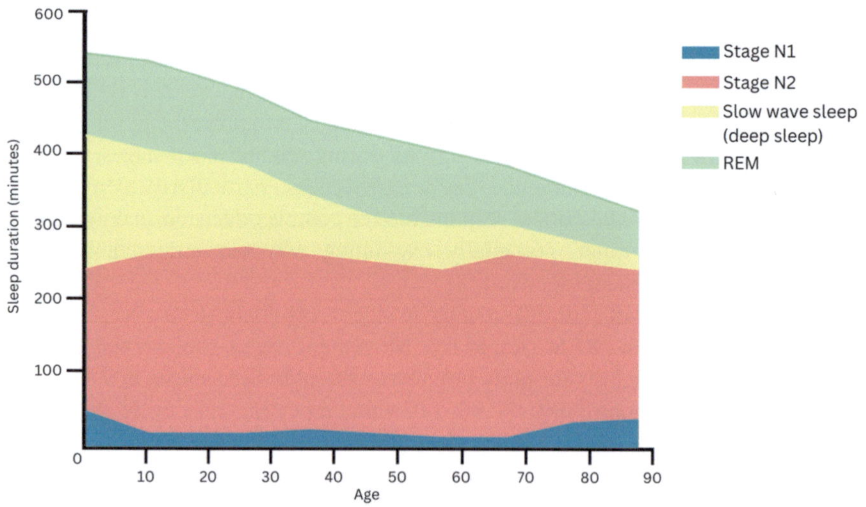

Fig. 2.1 How your sleep changes with age. ("Stacked area analysis was performed using GraphPad Prism version 10.4.1. for Windows, GraphPad Software, www.graphpad.com")

disrupted sleep [13]. These changing requirements align with developmental needs: infants' brains form millions of new neural connections every second in the first few years of life, and proper sleep is needed for development [14]. Teenagers, contrary to popular belief, aren't just being lazy when they sleep late—their biological sleep patterns naturally shift later so they feel sleepy later in the day and tend to wake up later, a phenomenon observed across cultures [15].

Sleep quality matters nearly as much as quantity, a fact that becomes increasingly clear as we age. Even if you do sleep 7–9 h, it does not mean you actually have quality sleep, i.e., cycling through sleep stages and spending an optimal time in each one to get the full benefits of restorative sleep. Scientists use the term "sleep hygiene"to describe practices that help optimize sleep [16]. Good sleep hygiene can lead to better sleep quality and improved daytime alertness. While avoiding caffeine, heavy meals, and alcohol near bedtime helps, sleep hygiene extends beyond simple rules. It encompasses creating an environment that promotes quality rest, from maintaining a cool, dark bedroom to following consistent sleep and wake times (very important!). The ideal bedroom temperature for sleep is around 19–20 °C (66–68 °F), as our body temperature naturally drops during sleep [17]. Regular physical activity and mindful eating patterns also play crucial roles in establishing healthy sleep patterns, though vigorous exercise should be avoided within 1-2 h of bedtime, as it can increase your sympathetic tone which is not helpful if you want to get some rest [18]. On the other hand, some studies show that evening exercise (more than 1 h before bedtime) may help people fall asleep faster and spend more time in deep sleep [19].

Sleep has its own architecture—an internal structure made up of four stages that repeat throughout the night [20] (Fig. 2.2). As mentioned earlier, these stages fall into two main categories: non-REM sleep (with three distinct stages: N1, N2, N3) and REM (Rapid Eye Movement) sleep. The journey begins with light sleep, known as Stage N1, where breathing slows and muscles start to relax. Brain waves begin to change, showing a pattern called theta waves on electroencephalography (EEG;

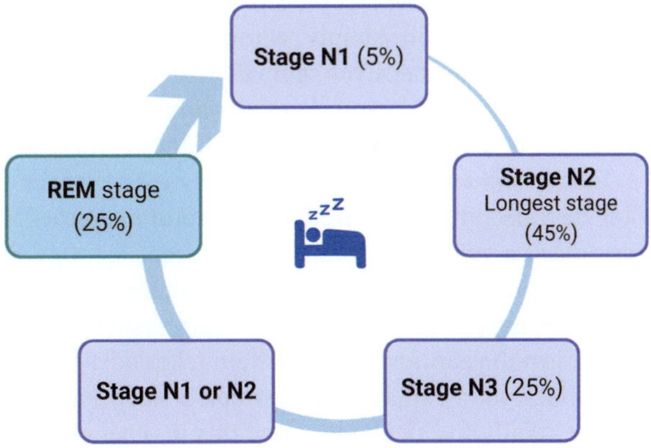

Fig. 2.2 The human sleep cycle pattern. ("Image generated by ChatGPT (OpenAI), 2025. Used with permission")

procedure to record brain activity using several electrodes places on the skull), which represent the boundary between wakefulness and sleep.

As you progress into Stage N2, your brain produces distinct EEG electrical patterns called sleep spindles and K-complexes [21]. These aren't just random electrical noise—they play vital roles in memory consolidation and protecting sleep from disruption. Your body temperature drops slightly, heart rate slows, and you become less aware of your surroundings. This stage typically occupies about 45% of total sleep time in adults, making it the most prevalent sleep stage [22].

Stage N3, or deep sleep, is the body's most restorative phase, ideally making up about 20% of total sleep time. The brain generates large, slow delta waves on EEG, and blood pressure and heart rate drop [20]. Growth hormone secretion peaks during this stage, promoting physical repair and regeneration [23]. The immune system becomes more active, explaining why adequate sleep helps fight off infections. Memory consolidation continues, but now focusing on procedural memories—physical skills and movements learned during the day [20].

REM sleep, which makes up about 20–25% of total sleep time, present a fascinating paradox: while the brain buzzes with activity similar to wakefulness, the body remains almost completely paralyzed [24]. This paralysis, called muscle atonia, prevents us from acting out our dreams [24]. During REM sleep, the brain processes emotional memories and experiences, helping us maintain psychological well-being. Dreams during REM sleep tend to be more vivid and story-like compared to the fragmentary dreams of other sleep stages. This stage also supports creative problem-solving, potentially explaining why solutions sometimes "come to us" after a good night's sleep.

Recent research has revealed sleep's crucial role in brain maintenance. During sleep, the space between brain cells actually increases, allowing for better circulation of cerebrospinal fluid [25]. This enhanced flow helps clear out metabolic waste products that accumulate during wakefulness, including proteins associated with neurodegenerative diseases like Alzheimer's disease [25]. This cleaning system, known as the glymphatic system, works efficiently during sleep, and especially during deep sleep.

The timing of sleep stages isn't random. Deep sleep dominates the early hours of the night, while REM sleep becomes more prevalent in the later hours [20]. This pattern appears consistently across mammals, suggesting its evolutionary but unknown importance. Even animals with unusual sleep patterns, like dolphins that sleep with one brain hemisphere at a time, show similar sleep stage characteristics, highlighting the fundamental nature of these processes [26, 27].

Sleep's influence extends into nearly every aspect of physical and mental function. The sleeping brain strengthens useful memories while pruning away unnecessary ones, a process essential for efficient learning. Hormonal regulation during sleep affects everything from appetite control to stress response. Growth and repair processes accelerate, while the immune system strengthens its ability to fight disease. Even the cardiovascular system takes advantage of sleep's restorative properties, which may explain why disrupted sleep increases the risk of cardiovascular disease. We'll dive deep into all of this in other chapters of the book.

References

1. Dang-Vu TT, Schabus M, Desseilles M, Sterpenich V, Bonjean M, Maquet P. Functional neuroimaging insights into the physiology of human sleep. Sleep. 2010;33(12):1589–603.
2. Ferrara M, Moroni F, De Gennaro L, Nobili L. Hippocampal sleep features: relations to human memory function. Front Neurol. 2012;3:57. PMID: 22529835.
3. Muzur A, Pace-Schott EF, Hobson JA. The prefrontal cortex in sleep. Trends Cogn Sci. 2002;6(11):475–81. PMID: 12457899.
4. Saper CB, Fuller PM, Pedersen NP, Lu J, Scammell TE. Sleep state switching. Neuron. 2010;68(6):1023–42. PMID: 21172606.
5. Rasch B, Born J. About sleep's role in memory. Physiol Rev. 2013;93(2):681–766. PMID: 23589831.
6. Elkhenany H, AlOkda A, El-Badawy A, El-Badri N. Tissue regeneration: impact of sleep on stem cell regenerative capacity. Life Sci. 2018;214:51–61. PMID: 30393021.
7. Besedovsky L, Lange T, Born J. Sleep and immune function. Pflugers Arch. 2012;463(1):121–137. PMID: 22071480.
8. Vandekerckhove M, Wang YL. Emotion, emotion regulation and sleep: an intimate relationship. AIMS Neurosci. 2017;5(1):1–17. PMID: 32341948.
9. Xie L, Kang H, Xu Q, Chen MJ, Liao Y, Thiyagarajan M, O'Donnell J, Christensen DJ, Nicholson C, Iliff JJ, Takano T, Deane R, Nedergaard M. Sleep drives metabolite clearance from the adult brain. Science. 2013;342(6156):373–7. PMID: 24136970.
10. Brooks PL, Peever JH. Identification of the transmitter and receptor mechanisms responsible for REM sleep paralysis. J Neurosci. 2012;32(29):9785–95. PMID: 22815493.
11. Watson NF, Badr MS, Belenky G, Bliwise DL, Buxton OM, Buysse D, Dinges DF, Gangwisch J, Grandner MA, Kushida C, Malhotra RK, Martin JL, Patel SR, Quan SF, Tasali E. Recommended amount of sleep for a healthy adult: a joint consensus statement of the American Academy of Sleep Medicine and Sleep Research Society. Sleep. 2015;38(6):843–4. PMID: 26039963.
12. Nevarez MD, Rifas-Shiman SL, Kleinman KP, Gillman MW, Taveras EM. Associations of early life risk factors with infant sleep duration. Acad Pediatr. 2010;10(3):187–93. PMID: 20347414.
13. Gulia KK, Kumar VM. Sleep disorders in the elderly: a growing challenge. Psychogeriatrics. 2018;18(3):155–65. PMID: 29878472
14. Center on the developing child at Harvard University. Brain architecture [Internet]. Cambridge, MA: Harvard University. Cited 2024 Dec 29. https://developingchild.harvard.edu/key-concept/brain-architecture
15. Hagenauer MH, Perryman JI, Lee TM, Carskadon MA. Adolescent changes in the homeostatic and circadian regulation of sleep. Dev Neurosci. 2009;31(4):276–84. PMID: 19546564.
16. Alanazi EM, Alanazi AMM, Albuhairy AH, Alanazi AAA. Sleep hygiene practices and its impact on mental health and functional performance among adults in Tabuk City: a cross-sectional study. Cureus. 2023;15(3):e36221. PMID: 37069886.
17. American Academy of Sleep Medicine. How to sleep better [Internet]. Darien: AASM. Cited 2024 Dec 28. https://aasm.org/resources/pdf/products/howtosleepbetter_web.pdf
18. Stutz J, Eiholzer R, Spengler CM. Effects of evening exercise on sleep in healthy participants: a systematic review and meta-analysis. Sports Med. 2019;49(2):269–87. PMID: 30374942.
19. Harvard Health Publishing. Does exercising at night affect sleep? [Internet]. Boston, MA: Harvard Medical School. Cited 2024 Dec 28. https://www.health.harvard.edu/staying-healthy/does-exercising-at-night-affect-sleep
20. Patel AK, Reddy V, Shumway KR, Araujo JF. Physiology, sleep stages. 2024 Jan 26. In: StatPearls [Internet]. Treasure Island: StatPearls; 2025 Jan–. PMID: 30252388.
21. Gandhi MH, Emmady PD. Physiology, K complex. 2023 May 1. In: StatPearls [Internet]. Treasure Island: StatPearls; 2025 Jan–. PMID: 32491401

22. Cleveland Clinic. Sleep [Internet]. Cleveland: Cleveland Clinic. Cited 2024 Dec 28. https://my.clevelandclinic.org/health/body/12148-sleep-basics
23. Zaffanello M, Pietrobelli A, Cavarzere P, Guzzo A, Antoniazzi F. Complex relationship between growth hormone and sleep in children: insights, discrepancies, and implications. Front Endocrinol (Lausanne). 2024;14:1332114. PMID: 38327902.
24. Feriante J, Araujo JF. Physiology, REM sleep. 2023 Feb 13. In: StatPearls [Internet]. Treasure Island: StatPearls Publishing; 2025 Jan–. PMID: 30285349
25. Chong PLH, Garic D, Shen MD, Lundgaard I, Schwichtenberg AJ. Sleep, cerebrospinal fluid, and the glymphatic system: a systematic review. Sleep Med Rev. 2022;61:101572. PMID: 34902819; PMCID.
26. Mascetti GG. Unihemispheric sleep and asymmetrical sleep: behavioral, neurophysiological, and functional perspectives. Nat Sci Sleep. 2016;8:221–238. https://doi.org/10.2147/NSS.S71970. Erratum in: Nat Sci Sleep 2016 Dec 20;9:1. PMID: 27471418.
27. Datta S. Cellular and chemical neuroscience of mammalian sleep. Sleep Med. 2010;11(5):431–440. PMID: 20359944.

The Circadian Rhythm

3

3.1 The Circadian Clock: Our Body's Internal Timekeeper

Within every living organism lies a biological timekeeper known as the circadian rhythm. This internal clock governs a 24-h cycle that controls fundamental aspects of our physiology, from sleep-wake patterns to hormone fluctuations and metabolic functions [1]. The scientific field dedicated to studying these biological rhythms, chronobiology, has revealed how these internal timekeepers regulate life's essential processes.

The discovery of internal rhythms traces back to 1729, when French scientist Jean-Jacques d'Ortous de Mairan conducted what would become a foundational experiment in chronobiology. While studying Mimosa plants, known for their daily leaf movements, de Mairan made a crucial observation: even when placed in complete darkness, the plants continued their daily pattern of folding leaves in the evening and opening them in the morning [2]. This simple yet profound experiment provided the first scientific evidence that living organisms possess an internal timing mechanism independent of external cues, in this case sunlight.

Over the next two centuries, scientists accumulated evidence that similar internal timing systems exist across the natural world, from single-celled organisms to humans. However, the molecular basis of these rhythms remained a mystery until the late twentieth century. The breakthrough came through research on tiny fruit flies, leading to the 2017 Nobel Prize in Physiology or Medicine awarded to Michael Young, Michael Rosbash, and Jeffrey Hall [3]. Their work revealed the fundamental molecular mechanisms controlling circadian rhythms, mechanisms later proven to be remarkably similar-though not identical-across many species.

The central circadian clock resides in the brain's hypothalamus, specifically within a group of approximately 20,000 neurons called the suprachiasmatic nucleus (SCN) [4]. This master clock's location is strategically important: it is located directly above the optic chiasm, where the optic nerves cross, allowing it to receive direct input from the eyes about environmental light conditions through a dedicated neural pathway from the retina called retinohypothalamic tract [5]. This anatomical positioning enables

A. Juginović, *Sleep Science Made Simple*,
https://doi.org/10.1007/978-3-031-92060-8_3

precise synchronization between our internal clock and the external environment, primarily through light—the most powerful cue for the SCN to determine it's day or night.

Light exposure plays a crucial role in maintaining proper circadian timing [6] (Fig. 3.1). When light hits specialized cells in our eye's retina called intrinsically photosensitive retinal ganglion cells (ipRGCs), they send signals directly to the SCN through the retinohypothalamic tract [6]. These cells are particularly sensitive to blue light, explaining why exposure to blue-rich LED screens on smartphones in the evening can disrupt our natural sleep timing. The SCN processes this light information and adjusts our internal clock accordingly, helping us stay synchronized with the external day-night cycle.

The molecular mechanism driving circadian rhythms in nearly every cell of our body relies on an elegant system of genetic feedback loops [7]. During daylight hours, two proteins in the cell, CLOCK and BMAL1, bind to specific sequences on the DNA in the cell nucleus, activating genes that produce two other key proteins: PERIOD (PER) and CRYPTOCHROME (CRY). These proteins reside, along with organelles like the mitochondria or ribosomes, in the cytoplasm which surrounds the cell nucleus. As these proteins accumulate throughout the day, they gradually form PER-CRY complexes that enter back into the cell nucleus. Once inside, they bind directly to the CLOCK and BMAL1 proteins. This binding stops CLOCK and BMAL1 from activating further production of PER and CRY proteins, effectively shutting down their own creation. This creates the self-regulating feedback loop that

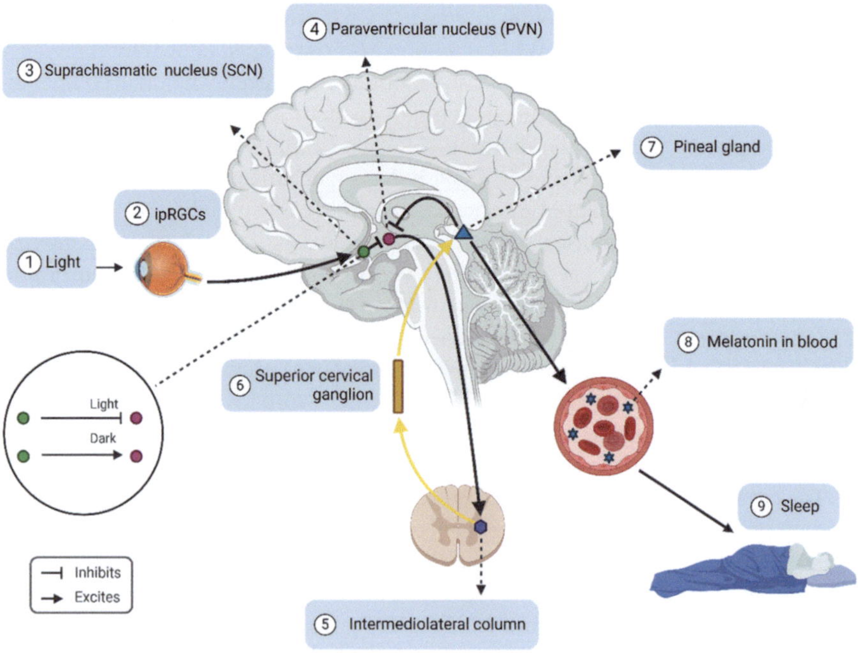

Fig. 3.1 Neural circuit of sleep-wake regulation. ("Created in BioRender. Juginovic, A. (2025) https://BioRender.com/u57d964")

takes about 24 h to complete, forming the foundation of our circadian rhythm (Fig. 3.2). While this explanation captures the core mechanism, the full process involves additional regulatory proteins and layers of control that further refine circadian timing.

The impact of circadian rhythms extends far beyond sleep and wakefulness [8]. These rhythms influence hormone production, body temperature regulation, metabolism, and even cognitive function. For example, cortisol, often called the "stress hormone," typically peaks in the early morning hours, helping prepare us for daily activities. Melatonin, a hormone crucial for initiating sleep, begins rising in the evening, peaks in the middle of the night, and gradually declines toward morning. Body temperature also follows a circadian pattern, dropping slightly during sleep and rising before awakening. Disrupting these natural rhythms—whether through irregular sleep schedules, shift work, or late-night screen use—can have serious health consequences. Studies show that chronic circadian disruption is linked to increased risk of obesity, diabetes, cardiovascular disease (e.g. stroke or heart attack), and mental health issues [9]. Even minor inconsistencies in sleep timing can impair memory formation, weaken immune function, and reduce cognitive performance [10, 11]. This is why maintaining a consistent sleep schedule, even on weekends, is crucial for optimal health. It keeps our internal clocks aligned with our body's natural rhythms, ensuring all these vital processes occur at their intended times.

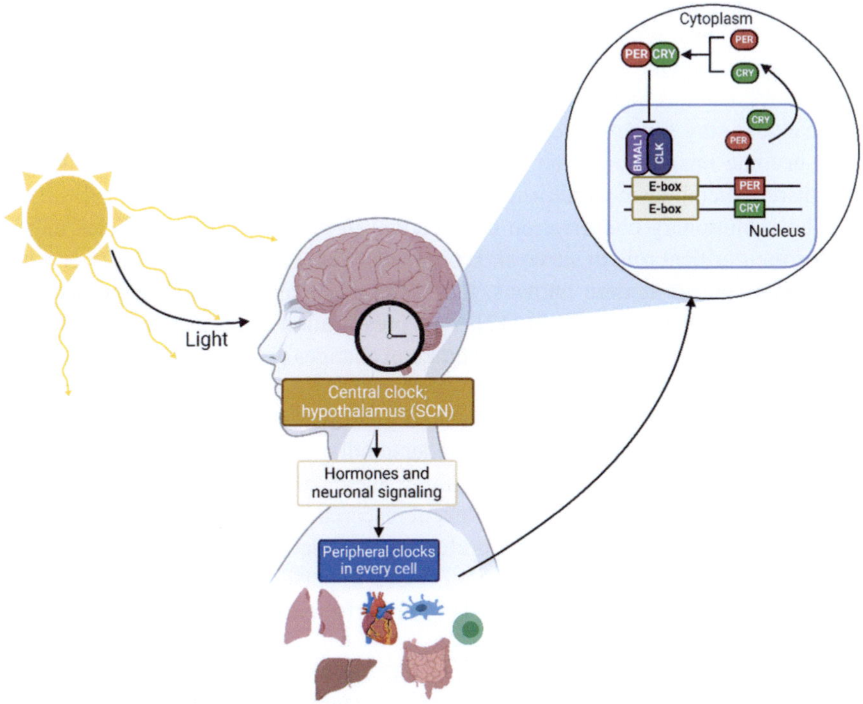

Fig. 3.2 Simplified molecular regulation of the circadian rhythm. ("Created in BioRender. Juginovic, A. (2025) https://BioRender.com/f03n895")

Circadian rhythms vary among individuals due to genetic differences in our biological clocks [12]. These variations create distinct chronotypes—natural preferences for when we feel most alert and when we prefer to sleep. "Morning larks" naturally wake early and are most productive in the morning hours, while "night owls" tend to be more alert in the evening and prefer later bedtimes [13]. Approximately 15–25% of people are morning types, 10–15% are evening types, and the majority fall somewhere in between—though these proportions can vary based on age, genetics, and environment. Although it's possible to adjust one's schedule, doing so against their chronotype may require extra effort and could negatively impact well-being. Research suggests that aligning our daily schedules—work, study, exercise—with our natural chronotype can improve performance, mood, and overall health. However, modern society, with its typical 9-to-5 schedule, often forces night owls to function against their natural rhythm, potentially contributing to what researchers call "social jet lag"[14]. This occurs when people must follow social or work schedules that conflict with their natural biological timing, similar to experiencing ongoing jet lag without ever traveling to a different time zone.

The central circadian clock in the brain (suprachiasmatic nucleus) also controls numerous peripheral clocks throughout the body [15]. These local timekeepers, found in nearly every cell in our body, help optimize organ function according to the time of day. The liver, for instance, increases its capacity for nutrient processing during our typical eating hours and shifts to energy storage during sleep. The heart adjusts its output and blood pressure in anticipation of daily activity, while muscles modify their sensitivity to insulin and energy utilization patterns. This hierarchical organization, with the SCN acting as the master clock coordinating multiple peripheral clocks, ensures that various biological processes occur at optimal times. When these clocks stay synchronized, our organs work efficiently and in harmony; when they become misaligned—due to irregular eating patterns or sleep schedules—it can disrupt metabolism, cardiovascular function, and long-term health [16].

The evolutionary conservation of circadian mechanisms across species underscores their critical role in survival. From cyanobacteria, which evolved over a billion years ago, to modern humans, the basic principles of circadian timing have remained remarkably consistent [17]. This preservation suggests that the ability to anticipate and prepare for daily environmental changes provides a significant evolutionary advantage.

The field of chronobiology continues to yield new insights into how circadian rhythms influence health and disease. Understanding these internal timekeepers has led to innovations in cancer treatment timing, medication scheduling, and strategies for managing jet lag and shift work. Recent research has even begun exploring how individual variations in circadian preferences—whether someone is naturally a "morning lark" or "night owl"—might be used to personalize health recommendations and optimize daily cognitive and motor performance.

Bonus Section: How Light Controls the Brain's Internal Clock. From Light to Brain: How Our Eyes Control Our Internal Clock—Optional Read (for those who want to learn even more).

3.1.1 How Light Controls the Brain's Internal Clock

The journey of how light regulates our biological clock begins in the eye, an organ whose complexity extends far beyond enabling vision. While most people understand eyes as instruments for seeing the world, they serve another essential function: synchronizing our internal clock with environmental light cycles. This dual purpose reflects millions of years of evolutionary refinement, resulting in an organ that not only creates images but also maintains our daily biological rhythms.

The process starts when light enters through the pupil and reaches the retina, a remarkably complex structure composed of ten distinct cellular layers [18]. Each layer serves specific functions in processing light information, making it one of the most sophisticated biological sensors known in nature. The retina contains the classic photoreceptors—rods for dim light vision and cones for color perception—but also houses a more recently discovered class of cells that revolutionized our understanding of circadian biology: the intrinsically photosensitive retinal ganglion cells (ipRGCs) [19].

The discovery of ipRGCs in the early 2000s solved a long-standing mystery in circadian biology. Scientists had observed that mice lacking both rods and cones—the traditional light-sensing cells—could still adjust their biological rhythms in response to light. This observation led to the identification of ipRGCs, a small population of cells that make up less than 5% of all ganglion cells in the retina [20]. These specialized neurons contain melanopsin, a light-sensitive protein that gives them the unique ability to detect environmental light levels independently of the classical photoreceptors.

Melanopsin's functions quite differently from the light-detecting proteins (photopigments) in rods and cones [21]. While traditional photoreceptors respond rapidly to light changes, allowing us to see moving objects and fine details, melanopsin responds more slowly and is particularly sensitive to blue light wavelengths around 480 nanometers—coincidentally matching the peak wavelength of daylight. This specialization makes ipRGCs perfectly suited for their role in circadian regulation. When light activates melanopsin in ipRGCs, it triggers a precise cascade of molecular events [21]. The process begins with a conformational change in the melanopsin protein, leading to the opening of ion channels in the cell membrane. This allows calcium ions to flow into the cell, creating an electrical signal that travels along the cell's axon. Unlike signals from conventional photoreceptors, which take multiple routes through the brain, these signals follow a dedicated pathway directly to the suprachiasmatic nucleus (SCN) in the brain's hypothalamus. As a reminder, the SCN is a group of around 20,000 neurons located just above where the optic nerves cross, and functions as the body's master clock, regulating sleep and wake cycles (Fig. 3.3).

This direct connection between ipRGCs and the SCN, known as the retinohypothalamic tract, represents a prime example of specialized neural wiring dedicated to circadian control [22]. The signals travel via the optic nerve but splits from the visual pathway at the optic chiasm, ensuring that circadian information reaches the

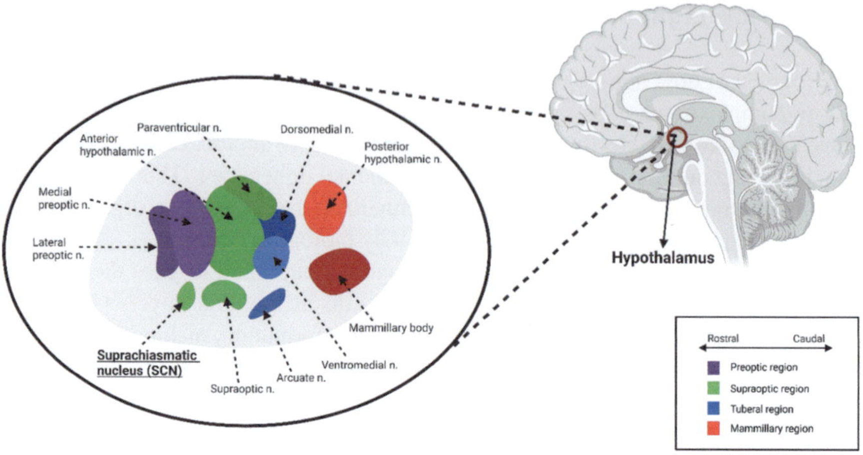

Fig. 3.3 Anatomical organization of the hypothalamus. ("Created in BioRender. Juginovic, A. (2025) https://BioRender.com/t75q493")

SCN without interference from image processing. When these signals arrive at the SCN, that initiates changes in the expression of circadian clock genes.

ipRGCs also receive input from rods and cones, enabling them to integrate overall brightness and spectral quality throughout the day. This integration enables our circadian system to respond both to the overall amount of environmental light and to subtle changes in light quality throughout the day. Morning light, rich in blue wavelengths, provides particularly strong signals to this system, explaining why morning light exposure is especially effective at reinforcing circadian alignment [23].

In our modern environment, this finely tuned system faces unprecedented challenges. Artificial lighting, particularly LED technology, can activate ipRGCs at inappropriate times, disrupting natural circadian rhythms. The blue light emitted by electronic devices is especially problematic because it closely matches the peak sensitivity of melanopsin [23]. Evening exposure to these devices can suppress melatonin release and delay the circadian phase, making it harder to fall asleep and maintain regular sleep patterns.

The critical role of this light-sensing system becomes particularly evident in studies of individuals with complete blindness. Research shows that most totally blind individuals experience significant circadian rhythm disruptions [24]. Without light input to their SCN, their internal clocks begin to "free-run," operating on cycles that may be longer or shorter than 24 h. These individuals often experience a condition called non-24-h sleep-wake rhythm disorder, causing their sleep-wake times to shift later each day.

Research with blind individuals has led to important therapeutic advances in circadian medicine. Studies have shown that carefully timed melatonin administration can help entrain sleep-wake cycles in both blind and sighted individuals with circadian disorders [25]. This work has also contributed to our understanding of how light therapy can be optimized for treating various circadian rhythm disruptions, from jet lag to shift work disorder.

Recent research has revealed additional complexity in how ipRGCs regulate circadian rhythms. These cells send signals not only to the SCN but also to other brain regions involved in mood, alertness, and cognitive function [26]. This broader influence helps explain why disrupted light exposure can affect not just sleep timing but also emotional well-being and cognitive performance.

3.1.2 Modern Life Versus Your Circadian Clock

Our internal clock requires consistent environmental cues to stay precisely aligned with the 24-h day. Scientists call these external time cues "zeitgebers," from the German word for "time givers"[27]. While various factors serve as zeitgebers—including temperature fluctuations, physical activity, and meal timing—light stands as the most powerful synchronizing agent. Research has shown that under natural conditions, our internal clock maintains a remarkably stable rhythm of approximately 24 h and 10 to 20 min, with typical individual variation of only about 15 min [12] (Fig. 3.4).

The crucial role of light in regulating biological rhythms was dramatically demonstrated in 1938 through a pioneering experiment. Scientists Nathaniel Kleitman and Bruce Richardson spent 32 days in Kentucky's Mammoth Cave in the United States, living in complete darkness, isolated from all natural light cues [28]. Without light to anchor their biological clocks, their sleep-wake cycles began to drift out of sync with the 24-h day. Their internal circadian period extended to 28 h [29]. This groundbreaking study revealed light's fundamental role in maintaining our daily rhythms and established the concept of "free-running" circadian rhythms—the natural period of our internal clock when isolated from external cues such as light.

The relationship between light and our circadian system involves various mechanisms that scientists have yet fully understood. Light's effects depend not just on

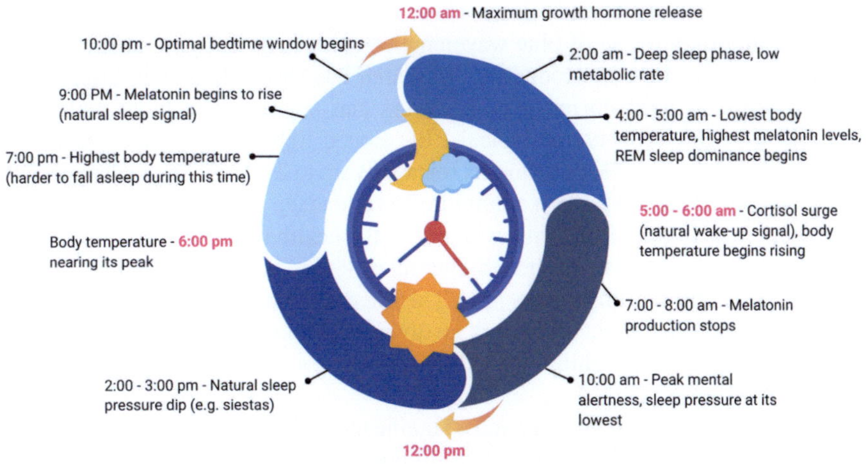

Fig. 3.4 Illustration of the body's biological clock across a 24-h day. ("Image generated by ChatGPT (OpenAI), 2025. Used with permission")

intensity but also on its spectral composition. Research has identified blue light, particularly wavelengths between 450 and 490 nanometers, as especially potent in regulating circadian rhythms [30]. This specific blue light is abundant in natural daylight but also comes from LED screens on our phones, tablets, and computers, as well as modern LED lighting. While natural daylight provides a balanced light spectrum, our digital screens and LED lights tend to emit a disproportionate amount of this biological clock-influencing blue light. During daylight hours, blue light exposure provides several benefits: it enhances alertness, improves cognitive performance, and positively affects mood through direct neural pathways from the retina to brain regions controlling these functions [31]. However, exposure to this same blue light in the evening can disrupt our natural sleep-wake cycle by suppressing melatonin production and shifting our internal clock later. This is particularly problematic in our modern world, where evening screen use has become routine, potentially contributing to widespread sleep problems and associated health issues.

The discovery of specialized retinal cells called intrinsically photosensitive retinal ganglion cells (ipRGCs) in the early 2000s revolutionized our understanding of how light affects circadian rhythms. Unlike conventional rod and cone photoreceptors used for vision, these cells contain melanopsin, a photopigment specifically tuned to detect environmental light levels [21]. These cells form direct neural connections to the brain's suprachiasmatic nucleus through the retinohypothalamic tract (explained in the previous section), allowing light information to rapidly influence our master clock.

When light strikes these specialized cells, they trigger a cascade of neural and hormonal responses. During daylight hours, this system promotes alertness by suppressing melatonin production and increasing cortisol levels [32]. As natural light fades in the evening, this suppression lifts, allowing melatonin levels to rise and prepare the body for sleep. This balance, refined over millions of years of evolution, faces unprecedented disruption in our modern environment. The widespread adoption of artificial lighting, particularly LED technology, has created novel challenges for human biology. These lights, especially those used in digital devices, emit high levels of blue wavelengths—precisely the type most effective at suppressing melatonin production. Research has shown that even brief exposure to artificial light during evening hours can significantly delay melatonin onset [33]. A 2-h exposure to typical LED screen light can suppress melatonin production by about 55%, delaying its release by up to 2 h [34]. The consequences of chronic circadian disruption extend far beyond sleep difficulties, as studies of shift workers provide compelling evidence of the health impacts of circadian misalignment. These individuals show higher rates of metabolic disorders, cardiovascular disease, and certain cancers [35]. The International Agency for Research on Cancer has classified night shift work involving circadian disruption as a probable human carcinogen, highlighting the seriousness of disturbed biological rhythms [36].

Shift work presents one of the most significant challenges to our circadian system. About 15–30% of the workforce in Europe and the United States work outside traditional daytime hours [37]. When people work at night under artificial lighting, their bodies receive contradictory signals: bright light tells the brain to stay alert while the internal clock signals sleep. This misalignment affects multiple body systems. Shift workers often experience not only disrupted sleep but also digestive problems, reduced immune function, and altered metabolism. Research shows they face higher risks of various health conditions, including cardiovascular disease, diabetes, and certain types of cancer [35].

Jet lag occurs when rapid travel across time zones creates a mismatch between our internal clock and the local time. A business traveler flying from Boston, MA, USA to Split, Croatia (my beautiful home town!) effectively forces their body to reset its entire biological rhythm by 6 h. This adjustment doesn't happen instantly—the body typically needs about 1 day per time zone crossed to fully adapt. Different body systems adjust at different rates, creating temporary chaos in our internal timing. The digestive system might be ready for dinner while the brain signals bedtime, resulting in the classic jet lag symptoms of fatigue, digestive issues, and sleep disruption [38].

"Social jet lag," a term coined by researchers, describes a common but less recognized form of circadian disruption [14]. This occurs when people maintain different schedules on workdays versus free days. This mismatch arises when weekday schedules force earlier wake times than one's natural preference. A person who wakes at 6 AM for work but sleeps until 9 AM on weekends essentially experiences a 3-h time zone shift every weekend. This misalignment between biological timing and social schedules can disrupt circadian rhythms and impact health, similar to regular jet lag but occurring without travel. Combined with modern habits—reduced exposure to natural daylight during work hours and increased evening exposure to artificial light from electronic devices—this misalignment can lead to chronic sleep debt and associated health risks.

In some cases, these natural timing preferences become extreme enough to qualify as circadian rhythm disorders (explained in detail in a separate later chapter) [39]. For example, delayed sleep phase disorder shifts sleep timing significantly later than conventional times, often by 2 h or more. Someone with this condition might naturally fall asleep at 3 AM and wake at 11 AM—a schedule that conflicts dramatically with typical work or school requirements. These patterns arise from a complex interaction between genetic factors, including variations in genes like PER2 and PER3, environmental influences, and age-related changes in circadian regulation [40].

Age affects our ability to handle circadian challenges [41]. Older adults often find it harder to adapt to shift work or recover from jet lag because their circadian systems become less flexible with age. In contrast, teenagers experience a natural evening delay in their circadian phase, conflicting with early school start times. This biological shift explains why forcing teenagers to wake early for school can significantly impact their learning and health.

Research into circadian mechanisms has revealed practical interventions for optimizing circadian health in the modern world. Timed light exposure—often referred to as chronotherapy—can realign the circadian clock and improve sleep patterns [42]. This involves maximizing natural light exposure in the morning, reducing blue light from screens in the evening using filters or apps, and creating a dark environment for sleep. The timing of these interventions is crucial: morning light has the strongest effect on reinforcing a healthy sleep-wake cycle, while avoiding bright light at night helps support the natural rise in melatonin levels. Beyond light-based strategies, chronotherapy also includes the timing of medication administration to align with biological rhythms, potentially enhancing treatment effectiveness and minimizing side effects, although there is still more research needed in this regard.

References

1. Reddy S, Reddy V, Sharma S. Physiology, circadian rhythm. In: StatPearls. Treasure Island (FL): StatPearls Publishing; 2025.
2. Ibáñez C. Discoveries of molecular mechanisms controlling the circadian rhythm. Stockholm: Nobel Prize Outreach AB; 2024. Available from: https://www.nobelprize.org/prizes/medicine/2017/advanced-information
3. The Nobel Prize. Press release. Stockholm: Nobel Prize Outreach AB; 2024. Available from: https://www.nobelprize.org/prizes/medicine/2017/press-release/
4. Ramkisoensing A, Meijer JH. Synchronization of biological clock neurons by light and peripheral feedback systems promotes circadian rhythms and health. Front Neurol. 2015;6:128.
5. Ma MA, Morrison EH. Neuroanatomy, nucleus suprachiasmatic. In: StatPearls [Internet]. Treasure Island (FL): StatPearls Publishing; 2025. Available from: https://www.ncbi.nlm.nih.gov/books/NBK546664/
6. LeGates TA, Fernandez DC, Hattar S. Light as a central modulator of circadian rhythms, sleep and affect. Nat Rev Neurosci. 2014;15(7):443–54.
7. Huang RC. The discoveries of molecular mechanisms for the circadian rhythm: the 2017 Nobel prize in physiology or medicine. Biom J. 2018;41(1):5–8. https://doi.org/10.1016/j.bj.2018.02.003.
8. Cleveland Clinic. Circadian rhythm. Cleveland: Cleveland Clinic; 2024. Available from: https://my.clevelandclinic.org/health/articles/circadian-rhythm
9. McHill AW, Hull JT, Klerman EB. Chronic circadian disruption and sleep restriction influence subjective hunger, appetite, and food preference. Nutrients. 2022;14(9):1800.
10. Zhang R, Tomasi D, Shokri-Kojori E, Wiers CE, Wang GJ, Volkow ND. Sleep inconsistency between weekends and weekdays is associated with changes in brain function during task and rest. Sleep. 2020;43(10):zsaa076.
11. Gooley JJ. How much day-to-day variability in sleep timing is unhealthy? Sleep. 2016;39(2):269–70.
12. Gentry NW, Ashbrook LH, Fu YH, Ptáček LJ. Human circadian variations. J Clin Invest. 2021;131(16):e148282.
13. Zhao C, He J, Xu H, Zhang J, Zhang G, Yu G. Are "night owls" or "morning larks" more likely to delay sleep due to problematic smartphone use? A cross-lagged study among undergraduates. Addict Behav. 2024;150:107906.
14. Wittmann M, Dinich J, Merrow M, Roenneberg T. Social jetlag: misalignment of biological and social time. Chronobiol Int. 2006;23(1–2):497–509.
15. Kowalska E, Brown SA. Peripheral clocks: keeping up with the master clock. Cold Spring Harb Symp Quant Biol. 2007;72:301–5.
16. Marino GM, Arble DM. Peripheral clock disruption and metabolic disease: moving beyond the anatomy to a functional approach. Front Endocrinol (Lausanne). 2023;14:1182506.
17. Demoulin CF, Lara YJ, Cornet L, François C, Baurain D, Wilmotte A, Javaux EJ. Cyanobacteria evolution: insight from the fossil record. Free Radic Biol Med. 2019;140:206–23.
18. Mahabadi N, Al Khalili Y. Neuroanatomy, Retina. [Updated 2023 Aug 8]. In: StatPearls [Internet]. Treasure Island (FL): StatPearls Publishing; 2025. Available from: https://www.ncbi.nlm.nih.gov/books/NBK545310/

19. Pickard GE, Sollars PJ. Intrinsically photosensitive retinal ganglion cells. Rev Physiol Biochem Pharmacol. 2012;162:59–90.
20. Graham DM, Wong KY. Melanopsin-expressing, intrinsically photosensitive retinal ganglion cells (ipRGCs). In: Kolb H, Fernandez E, Jones B, Nelson R, editors. Webvision: the organization of the retina and visual system. Salt Lake City: University of Utah Health Sciences Center; 1995.
21. Do MTH. Melanopsin and the intrinsically photosensitive retinal ganglion cells: biophysics to behavior. Neuron. 2019;104(2):205–26.
22. Gooley JJ, Lu J, Chou TC, Scammell TE, Saper CB. Melanopsin in cells of origin of the retinohypothalamic tract. Nat Neurosci. 2001;4(12):1165.
23. Ziółkowska N, Chmielewska-Krzesinska M, Vyniarska A, Sienkiewicz W. Exposure to blue light reduces Melanopsin expression in intrinsically photoreceptive retinal ganglion cells and damages the inner retina in rats. Invest Ophthalmol Vis Sci. 2022;63(1):26.
24. Sack RL, Lewy AJ, Blood ML, Keith LD, Nakagawa H. Circadian rhythm abnormalities in totally blind people: incidence and clinical significance. J Clin Endocrinol Metab. 1992;75(1):127–34.
25. Sack RL, Brandes RW, Kendall AR, Lewy AJ. Entrainment of free-running circadian rhythms by melatonin in blind people. N Engl J Med. 2000;343(15):1070–7.
26. Maruani J, Geoffroy PA. Multi-level processes and retina-brain pathways of photic regulation of mood. J Clin Med. 2022;11(2):448.
27. Quante M, Mariani S, Weng J, Marinac CR, Kaplan ER, Rueschman M, Mitchell JA, James P, Hipp JA, Cespedes Feliciano EM, Wang R, Redline S. Zeitgebers and their association with rest-activity patterns. Chronobiol Int. 2019;36(2):203–13.
28. Martin C. Sleep is the best medicine. BMJ. 2007;335(7631):1216.
29. University of Chicago Library. Mammoth Cave. Chicago: University of Chicago; 2024. Available from: https://www.lib.uchicago.edu/collex/exhibits/discovering-beauty/mammoth-cave/?t
30. Moore-Ede M, Heitmann A. Circadian potency Spectrum in light-adapted humans. J Cell Sci Ther. 2022;13(5):361.
31. Alkozei A, Smith R, Pisner DA, Vanuk JR, Berryhill SM, Fridman A, Shane BR, Knight SA, Killgore WD. Exposure to blue light increases subsequent functional activation of the prefrontal cortex during performance of a working memory task. Sleep. 2016;39:1671.
32. Kim TW, Jeong JH, Hong SC. The impact of sleep and circadian disturbance on hormones and metabolism. Int J Endocrinol. 2015;2015:1.
33. Burgess HJ, Molina TA. Home lighting before usual bedtime impacts circadian timing: a field study. Photochem Photobiol. 2014;90:723.
34. Alam M, Abbas K, Sharf Y, Khan S. Impacts of blue light exposure from electronic devices on circadian rhythm and sleep disruption in adolescent and young adult students. Chronobiol Med. 2024;6(1):10–4.
35. Roth JR, Varshney S, de Moraes RCM, Melkani GC. Circadian-mediated regulation of cardiometabolic disorders and aging with time-restricted feeding. Obesity (Silver Spring). 2023;31(Suppl 1):40–9.
36. Erren TC, Falaturi P, Morfeld P, Knauth P, Reiter RJ, Piekarski C. Shift work and cancer: the evidence and the challenge. Dtsch Arztebl Int. 2010;107(38):657–62.
37. Wu QJ, Sun H, Wen ZY, Zhang M, Wang HY, He XH, Jiang YT, Zhao YH. Shift work and health outcomes: an umbrella review of systematic reviews and meta-analyses of epidemiological studies. J Clin Sleep Med. 2022;18(2):653–62.
38. Sack RL. The pathophysiology of jet lag. Travel Med Infect Dis. 2009;7(2):102–10.
39. Reid KJ, Zee PC. Circadian rhythm disorders. Semin Neurol. 2009;29(4):393–405.
40. Plavc L, Skubic C, Dolenc Grošelj L, Rozman D. Variants in the circadian clock genes *PER2* and *PER3* associate with familial sleep phase disorders. Chronobiol Int. 2024;41(5):757–66.
41. Duffy JF, Zitting KM, Chinoy ED. Aging and circadian rhythms. Sleep Med Clin. 2015;10(4):423–34.
42. Cardinali DP, Brown GM, Pandi-Perumal SR. Chronotherapy. Handb Clin Neurol. 2021;179:357–70.

Sleep Labs: How We Study Sleep

4

4.1 The Tools We Use to Study Sleep

The science of sleep relies on sophisticated tools to understand what happens in our brains and bodies during the night. These diagnostic methods help sleep doctors identify sleep disorders and determine the best treatments for their patients.

One of our most important tools is electroencephalography or EEG [1]. This technique measures the electrical activity produced by our brains using small electrodes placed on specific points of the scalp. These electrodes detect tiny voltage changes—measured in millionths of a volt—that reflect the synchronized activity of a group of brain cells. When displayed on a computer screen, these signals create distinctive wave patterns that tell us what stage of sleep someone has entered. However, EEG has its limitations—it only captures activity near the brain's surface, missing deeper brain regions that play important roles in sleep regulation. Even with these limitations, it offers very valuable insights that help the medical staff determine each sleep stage.

The gold standard for diagnosing sleep disorders is polysomnography—a comprehensive overnight sleep study that records multiple aspects of sleep simultaneously (Fig. 4.1) [1].

During polysomnography, patients spend the night in a sleep clinic while connected to various monitoring devices. Beyond brain waves, these devices track:

- Eye movements.
- Muscle activity.
- Heart rhythm.
- Breathing patterns.
- Blood oxygen levels.
- Body position.

A. Juginović, *Sleep Science Made Simple*,
https://doi.org/10.1007/978-3-031-92060-8_4

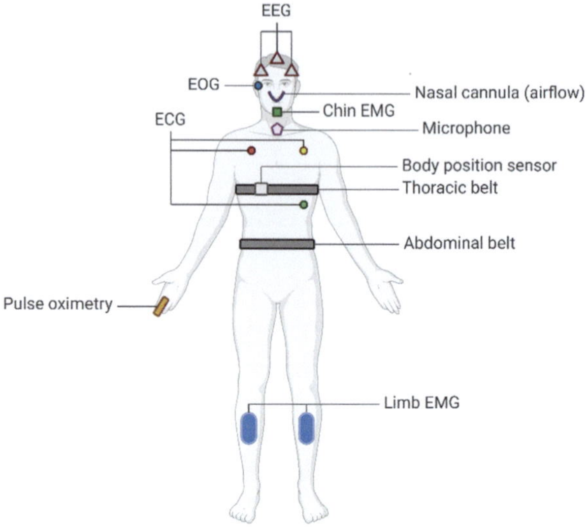

Fig. 4.1 Standard sleep study equipment (Polysomnography). ("Created in BioRender. Juginovic, A. (2025) https://BioRender.com/b30w055")

This wealth of information allows sleep specialists to create a detailed map of sleep called a hypnogram, showing how someone moves through different sleep stages throughout the night. This helps identify disruptions in normal sleep patterns and diagnose specific sleep disorders (Fig. 4.2).

For some sleep problems, particularly breathing disorders like sleep apnea, doctors might recommend a simpler test called polygraphy [2]. Unlike polysomnography, this test doesn't measure brain waves but focuses on breathing, heart rate, and oxygen levels. A major advantage of polygraphy is that patients can sleep in their own beds, as the monitoring equipment is portable and can be set up at home. In contrast, setting up an EEG (part of polysomnography) independently is very difficult.

One interesting challenge in sleep testing involves what scientists call the "First Night Effect" [3]. When people sleep in an unfamiliar environment like a sleep clinic, their sleep patterns often change. Some people sleep worse than usual due to anxiety about the strange surroundings or discomfort with the monitoring equipment. Others, surprisingly, might sleep better than normal, perhaps because they feel reassured by the medical supervision. This effect can complicate the interpretation of sleep studies, which is why sleep specialists always consider this factor when evaluating results.

Advances in sleep monitoring technology continue to improve our understanding of sleep. Modern systems can process multiple data streams in real time, helping identify subtle patterns that might indicate specific sleep disorders. This technology, combined with experienced medical interpretation, helps ensure accurate diagnosis and appropriate treatment for the millions of people affected by sleep disorders.

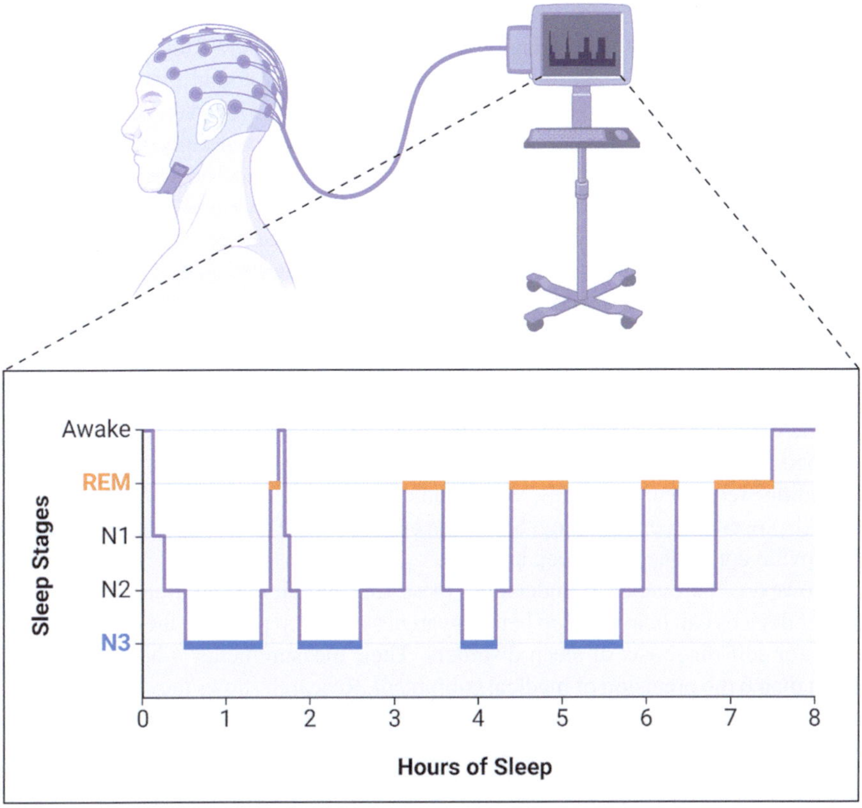

Fig. 4.2 Sleep stage distribution through the night. ("Created in BioRender. Juginovic, A. (2025) https://BioRender.com/k07m798")

4.1.1 Consumer Sleep Tech: Innovations and Current Challenges

While medical sleep studies remain the gold standard for diagnosing sleep disorders, recent years have seen remarkable advances in consumer devices that track and analyze sleep. These technologies offer individuals yet unprecedented insight into their nightly rest, though their capabilities and limitations deserve careful consideration [4].

Modern wearable devices use sophisticated combinations of sensors to estimate sleep patterns. Most rely on accelerometers to detect movement, along with heart rate sensors and temperature monitors. Some newer devices even incorporate blood oxygen monitoring—a measurement traditionally reserved for medical equipment. These devices analyze multiple data streams simultaneously to create detailed pictures of sleep architecture [4].

The accuracy of these devices continues to improve, as demonstrated by recent research. A 2024 study comparing three popular devices (Oura Ring, Fitbit Sense 2, and Apple Watch Series 8) to clinical polysomnography found they could detect sleep versus wake states with around 95% accuracy [5]. However, their ability to distinguish between different sleep stages proved more variable, with accuracy ranging from 50% to around 75% depending on the device and sleep stage being measured [5]. While not ideal, technology is still progressing at a rapid pace and may reach levels comparable to traditional polysomnography.

Smart mattresses represent another emerging category in sleep technology [6]. These high-tech beds incorporate pressure sensors and temperature regulation systems throughout their surface to track movement, breathing patterns, and sometimes heart rate. Many can automatically adjust firmness and temperature based on sleep data, though research validating their effectiveness remains relatively limited.

The explosion of sleep apps has also transformed how people approach sleep. Beyond basic alarm functions, modern sleep apps offer sophisticated features including sleep sound libraries, smart home integration for environmental control, and AI-powered sleep coaching. Some can even integrate data from multiple sources to provide comprehensive sleep analysis.

However, it's crucial to understand these technologies' limitations. While consumer devices can help develop better awareness of sleep patterns, they shouldn't be used for self-diagnosis of sleep disorders. Their measurements, while interesting, don't match the precision of medical equipment. Research shows they tend to under- or over-estimate sleep time and can't reliably distinguish between all sleep stages with medical accuracy. In fact, over-reliance on these devices can even lead to orthosomnia, a condition where individuals become excessively preoccupied with achieving perfect sleep, leading to increased stress and anxiety.

Looking ahead, sleep technology continues to advance rapidly. Newer devices incorporate artificial intelligence to analyze sleep patterns and provide increasingly personalized recommendations. Some can integrate with smart home systems to automatically optimize bedroom conditions throughout the night. While these innovations show promise, the fundamental principles of good sleep hygiene—consistent schedules, proper sleep environment, and healthy sleep habits—remain more important than any technology. Remember that good sleep doesn't require technology—many people sleep perfectly well without tracking devices. However, for those interested in understanding their sleep patterns better, modern sleep technology can provide valuable insights when used appropriately and with realistic expectations about its capabilities.

References

1. Rundo JV, Downey R 3rd. Polysomnography. Handb Clin Neurol. 2019;160:381–92.
2. Chiner E, Cánovas C, Molina V, Sancho-Chust JN, Vañes S, Pastor E, Martinez-Garcia MA. Home respiratory polygraphy is useful in the diagnosis of childhood obstructive sleep apnea syndrome. J Clin Med. 2020;9(7):2067.

3. Hu S, Shi L, Li Z, Ma Y, Li J, Bao Y, Lu L, Sun H. First-night effect in insomnia disorder: a systematic review and meta-analysis of polysomnographic findings. J Sleep Res. 2024;33(1):e13942.
4. de Zambotti M, Goldstein C, Cook J, Menghini L, Altini M, Cheng P, Robillard R. State of the science and recommendations for using wearable technology in sleep and circadian research. Sleep. 2024;47(4):zsad325.
5. Robbins R, Weaver MD, Sullivan JP, Quan SF, Gilmore K, Shaw S, Benz A, Qadri S, Barger LK, Czeisler CA, Duffy JF. Accuracy of three commercial wearable devices for sleep tracking in healthy adults. Sensors (Basel). 2024;24(20):6532.
6. Zhang Z, Jin X, Wan Z, Zhu M, Wu S. A feasibility study on smart mattresses to improve sleep quality. J Healthc Eng. 2021;2021:6127894.

Inside the Sleeping Brain: From Chemistry to Dreams

5

5.1 Brain at Night: Molecular and Electrical Foundations of Sleep and Its Stages

5.1.1 The Molecular Mechanisms Behind Our Brain's Transition from Wake to Sleep

Falling asleep each day is regulated by two key biological systems: Process S and Process C. Process S builds up sleep pressure—the longer we stay awake, the more our need for sleep increases. Process C reflects our internal 24-h circadian clock, or circadian rhythm, which regulates when we naturally feel awake or sleepy [1]. Together, these processes explain why we get more tired the longer we stay up and why we feel sleepy at night, even if we've napped during the day.

Process S primarily operates through a molecule called adenosine [1]. As we use energy throughout our waking hours, adenosine gradually builds up in the brain, acting as a natural sleep signal. Whenever our brain cells use energy—whether for thinking, movement, or simply staying awake—they break down the "energy molecule" ATP (adenosine triphosphate), which can lead to the release and accumulation of adenosine, a key factor in promoting sleepiness. This buildup creates increasing pressure to sleep, explaining why staying awake becomes progressively more difficult as the day goes on. During sleep, the brain clears away this accumulated adenosine, which is why we feel refreshed after a good night's rest.

Adenosine affects several key brain regions to promote sleep [2]. In areas like the basal forebrain and pons, it binds to specific receptors (A1 receptors) on neurons that normally keep us alert by releasing a neurotransmitter called acetylcholine. When adenosine attaches to these neurons, it reduces their activity, promoting drowsiness. This mechanism helps explain why caffeine keeps us awake—it blocks these same A1 receptors, preventing adenosine from delivering its "sleep signal".

The brain's wake-promoting system includes special neurons in the hypothalamus that produce a chemical called hypocretin (also known as orexin) [3]. These neurons play such a vital role in maintaining wakefulness that their loss leads to narcolepsy,

A. Juginović, *Sleep Science Made Simple*,
https://doi.org/10.1007/978-3-031-92060-8_5

a condition where people feel extremely sleepy during the day and can even fall asleep uncontrollably. This loss of hypocretin-producing neurons, often due to an autoimmune response, affects roughly 1 in 2000 people [4]. As adenosine levels rise throughout the day, it suppresses these neurons, further promoting the transition to sleep. This suppression occurs alongside other changes in the brain, including decreased activity in wake-promoting regions like the ascending reticular activating system (ARAS) in the brainstem and reduced levels of other alertness-promoting neurotransmitters such as norepinephrine and histamine. The coordinated reduction in wake-promoting activity, combined with the activation of sleep-promoting regions, helps ensure a smooth transition from wakefulness to sleep (Fig. 5.1).

Meanwhile, adenosine also activates sleep-promoting neurons in a region called the ventrolateral preoptic nucleus (VLPO), located in the anterior hypothalamus near the base of the brain [5]. These neurons release GABA, the brain's primary inhibitory chemical. Think of GABA as the brain's primary "quiet down" signal, reducing the activity of wake-promoting systems throughout the brain. This process resembles systematically dimming the lights throughout a house, as each wake-promoting system gradually powers down.

Working in parallel with the adenosine-driven sleep pressure (Process S), Process C—our circadian rhythm—helps explain why we feel sleepy at night even after you've taken a late-afternoon nap [1]. While adenosine accumulation creates direct sleep pressure, the brain's master clock, located in the suprachiasmatic nucleus, simultaneously controls this daily timing system, i.e., our 24-h rhythm. Each evening, it signals the pineal gland to begin producing melatonin, often called the "sleep hormone". Melatonin levels start rising in the evening, peak in the middle of the night, and decrease toward morning, helping regulate our sleep-wake cycle. These two processes—sleep pressure and circadian rhythm—operate simultaneously but independently, creating a sophisticated dual control system for sleep regulation.

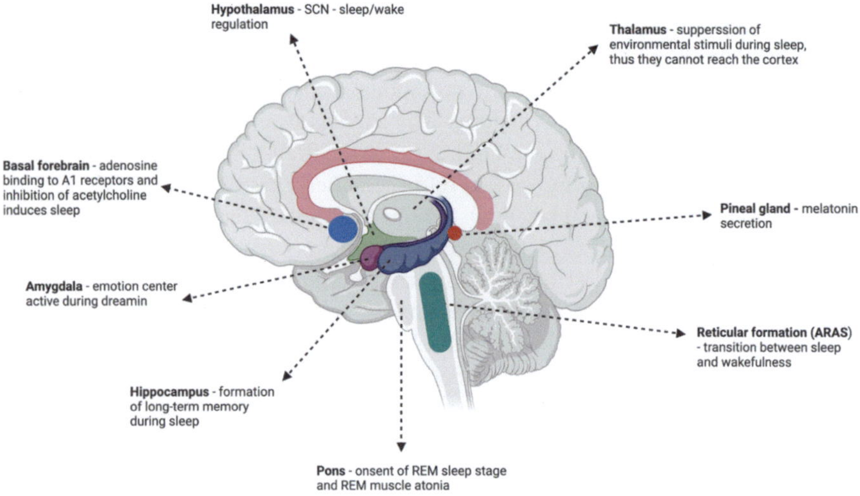

Fig. 5.1 Key brain regions involved in sleep regulation. ("Created in BioRender. Juginovic, A. (2025) https://BioRender.com/y91d094")

The brain maintains wakefulness through a network called the ascending reticular activating system (ARAS) [6]. This system keeps the brain alert and responsive during waking hours, like a sentinel that maintains alertness and awareness. Originating in the brainstem, the ARAS extends upward, influencing the thalamus, hypothalamus, and cerebral cortex. It uses various neurotransmitters—including norepinephrine, acetylcholine, histamine, and dopamine—to regulate wakefulness and maintain arousal. Each of these neurotransmitters plays a specific role in wakefulness, though they have many other functions throughout the brain and body. Norepinephrine enhances alertness and attention, acetylcholine supports cognitive function and awareness, histamine promotes general wakefulness, and dopamine contributes to motivation and reward-based arousal [7]. The ARAS also receives input from sensory systems, helping us stay responsive to important environmental cues, such as a baby's cry or an alarm clock. As we transition to sleep, sleep-promoting neurons inhibit this system, gradually reducing our awareness of our surroundings. This inhibition occurs in stages, with different ARAS components powering down in sequence—similar to shutting down a complex machine one circuit at a time. As a result, external sounds and movements become less likely to disturb us in deeper sleep, though the brain retains the ability to detect critical stimuli—an evolutionary adaptation that helped protect our ancestors while they slept.

These molecular mechanisms have important practical implications. For instance, while melatonin supplements can help adjust sleep timing in certain situations (such as jet lag or shift work), they represent only one aspect of the sleep-regulation system. A melatonin pill can signal "nighttime" to your brain, but it cannot override a build-up of wake-promoting signals or compensate for poor sleep habits. Similarly, caffeine can block adenosine receptors to promote wakefulness, but it doesn't eliminate the underlying sleep pressure—which explains why people often experience a "crash" when the effects of caffeine wear off. Quality sleep typically requires proper sleep habits and environment, as these brain mechanisms work best with consistent schedules and appropriate sleeping conditions. This means maintaining regular sleep-wake times, creating a dark and quiet sleep environment, avoiding evening screen exposure (which can suppress natural melatonin production), and allowing enough time for both Process S and Process C to operate optimally. Understanding these mechanisms helps explain why shortcuts to better sleep often prove ineffective in the long run, and why sustainable improvements usually require aligning our habits with our brain's natural sleep-regulatory systems.

Modern life can significantly impact these natural sleep processes. Evening exposure to bright lights, especially the blue light from electronic devices, can suppress melatonin production. Irregular sleep schedules can confuse our circadian timing system. Stress and anxiety can activate wake-promoting brain regions, making it harder to fall asleep even when adenosine levels are high. Even diet affects sleep—caffeine's ability to block adenosine receptors explains why that late afternoon coffee might keep you awake at night.

These mechanisms explain many common sleep experiences. That intense sleepiness after a long day? That's the effect of accumulated adenosine. The alertness you feel after waking from a good night's sleep? That's your wake-promoting systems reactivating in a brain cleared of sleep-inducing chemicals. The drowsiness that hits around the same time each evening? That's your circadian system releasing melatonin on schedule.

5.1.2 The Temperature-Sleep Connection: How Body Temperature Affects Our Rest

Our body temperature follows a precise 24-h pattern that profoundly influences sleep [8]. This temperature rhythm, refined over millions of years of evolution, helps control our daily cycles of alertness and sleepiness. Throughout the day, our core body temperature fluctuates by about 1 °C (1.8 °F), typically peaking in the late afternoon and reaching its lowest point in the early morning hours, around 3–5 AM (Fig. 5.2).

The process of falling asleep requires a decrease in core body temperature. This cooling mechanism involves an interesting biological process. Blood vessels near the skin's surface—in areas like our hands, feet, and face—begin to expand (dilate), a process called peripheral vasodilation [8]. This dilation is triggered in part by reduced its production of noradrenaline, a hormone that normally keeps blood vessels constricted. As these blood vessels dilate, they allow more blood to flow to the skin's surface, effectively transferring heat from our body's core to its exterior.

This heat transfer creates an interesting paradox: while our core temperature drops, our hands and feet actually warm up. Think of it like a car's radiator system—the engine (our core) cools down by transferring heat to the radiator (our skin), which then releases this heat to the surrounding environment. This explains why many people experience warm hands and feet just before falling asleep.

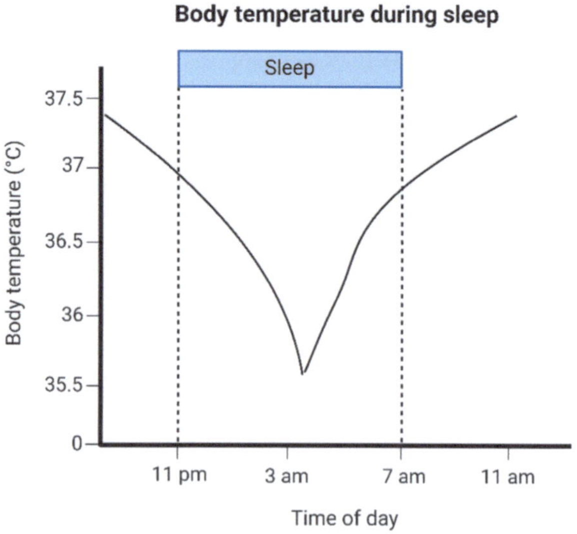

Fig. 5.2 Body temperature during sleep. ("Created in BioRender. Juginovic, A. (2025) https://BioRender.com/n99v409")

During sleep, our core temperature drops by about 1–1.30 °C (1.8–2.3 °F) [8]. This reduction isn't just a passive consequence of sleep—it actively promotes various restorative processes. The cooler body temperature slows metabolism, reduces energy consumption, and facilitates the repair and restoration of tissues. Even after we fall asleep, our core temperature continues to drop while skin temperature remains relatively warm, maintaining a temperature difference that helps preserve sleep.

The relationship between temperature and melatonin shows remarkable precision. As evening approaches, the body begins producing melatonin. This increase in melatonin coincides with the start of core temperature decline. When our core temperature reaches its lowest point in the early morning hours, melatonin levels peak [9]. This synchronization between temperature and melatonin helps ensure proper sleep timing and quality.

Research has revealed practical applications of this temperature-sleep connection. Taking a warm bath or shower 1–2 h before bedtime can improve sleep quality [10]. The warm water causes blood vessels near the skin to dilate, promoting heat loss from the core—similar to how a car's engine continues cooling even after being turned off. This explains why a warm bath makes many people feel sleepy.

Exercise timing also affects this temperature-sleep relationship [11]. Physical activity temporarily raises core body temperature, which can interfere with sleep if performed too close to bedtime. However, as the body cools after exercise, this post-exercise temperature drop can promote sleepiness. This explains why experts often recommend completing vigorous exercise at least 1–2 h before bedtime, allowing enough time for proper cooling.

The optimal bedroom temperature for sleep falls between 18 °C and 19 °C (66–68 °F) [12]. This range promotes the core temperature drop necessary for good sleep while preventing excessive heat loss that might cause discomfort. Higher room temperatures can interfere with this natural cooling process, making it harder to fall and stay asleep.

Bedding choices also play a significant role in temperature regulation during sleep. Materials that trap too much heat can prevent proper core temperature reduction, while breathable fabrics allow better temperature regulation. This explains why many people sleep better with layered bedding they can adjust throughout the night as their temperature needs change.

Temperature sensitivity varies throughout the night and across different sleep stages. During REM sleep, our body's ability to regulate temperature decreases and our temperature is more influenced by our environment [13]. This makes maintaining a consistent, cool room temperature particularly important for quality REM sleep. New mattress materials and climate control systems aim to optimize sleep by maintaining ideal temperature conditions throughout the night. Some cooling systems even adjust temperatures gradually to match our body's natural temperature rhythm, potentially promoting deeper and more restful sleep.

5.1.3 Understanding the Stages of Sleep

When we're awake, our brain exhibits distinct patterns of electrical activity that reflect our level of awareness and engagement with the world around us. This waking state allows us to think, move, and interact with our environment. During active, focused attention, the brain produces rapid electrical patterns called beta waves, oscillating 16–31 times per second [14]. When we're relaxed but still awake, these patterns shift to slightly slower alpha waves, particularly in the back of the brain. As a reminder, brain activity is tracked using electroencephalography (EEG), a technique that records the brain's electrical signals from the scalp using electrodes.

As we begin to fall asleep, brain activity follows a predictable sequence of changes (Fig. 5.3). Think of it as your brain gradually turning down its activity level, like slowly dimming the lights in a room. As drowsiness begins, the crisp, fast patterns of wakefulness start to fade. The brain transitions into sleep stage N1, where slower theta waves emerge, marking the beginning of sleep [14]. This transition often feels familiar to anyone who has caught themselves nodding off while reading or watching television.

As sleep deepens, the brain's electrical patterns continue to change dramatically. The waves become increasingly larger and slower, particularly during deep sleep (stage N3), where powerful delta waves dominate [14]. These slow waves reflect the brain's shift into its most restorative state. When REM sleep begins, the brain's electrical activity resembles that of wakefulness, despite the person being deeply asleep [14]. This peculiar pattern, along with increased heart rate and breathing, led scientists to call REM sleep "paradoxical sleep"—the EEG resembles wakefulness, while the person remains deeply asleep and physically immobile.

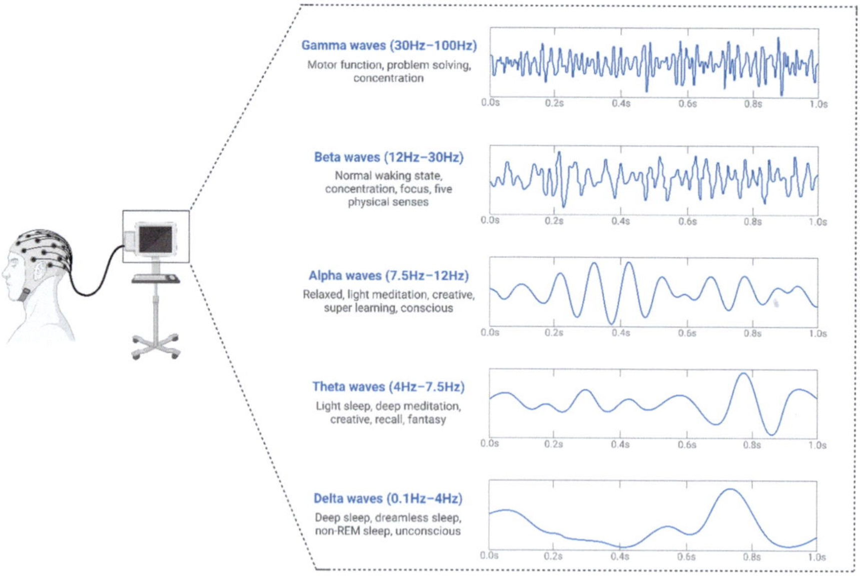

Fig. 5.3 Types of brain wave activity. ("Created in BioRender. Juginovic, A. (2025) https://BioRender.com/q69f078")

These changes in brain activity correspond with broader changes throughout the body. As sleep progresses, muscles gradually relax, reaching their most relaxed state during REM sleep, when most muscles become temporarily paralyzed. This natural paralysis prevents us from acting out our dreams. Eye movements also follow a distinct pattern—they slow down as sleep deepens, only to burst into periodic rapid movements during REM sleep, giving this stage its name.

The body's automatic functions also shift during sleep [15]. The parasympathetic nervous system—responsible for "rest and digest" functions—becomes more active during non-REM sleep, leading to slower, more regular breathing and heart rate. During REM sleep, however, the sympathetic nervous system—our "fight or flight" system—becomes intermittently more active, contributing to variability in heart rate and blood pressure. This activation of the sympathetic nervous system, particularly in the early morning hours, helps explain why heart attacks occur more frequently during this time.

These complex changes in brain activity and body function during sleep weren't easy to discover. Scientists like Hans Berger, who developed the first human electroencephalogram (EEG) in the 1920s to detect brain activity, pioneered our ability to measure and understand brain activity during sleep [16]. The alpha waves he first identified during relaxed wakefulness (now sometimes called "Berger's waves" in his honor) marked the beginning of our ability to scientifically study sleep.

These patterns reveal why sleep can't simply switch on and off like a light—it's a gradual process of the brain and body transitioning through different states. This insight has practical implications for why activities like meditation or relaxation exercises can help prepare the brain for sleep, and why suddenly waking from deep sleep can leave us feeling groggy and disoriented. Let's explore each stage of sleep, one by one.

5.1.3.1 Stage N1 Sleep: Light and Short

As we begin to drift off to sleep, our brain enters its first sleep stage, known as N1. This initial phase represents our lightest form of sleep—a transitional state between wakefulness and deeper sleep where we hover at the edge of consciousness [17]. During this time, our brain waves begin to slow down, shifting from the rapid patterns of wakefulness to gentler, slower waves called theta waves.

Think of N1 sleep as wading into the shallow end of a pool—you're in the water, but you can easily step back onto dry land. During this stage, which typically makes up about 5% of our total sleep time, we can be awakened by a quiet noise, a light touch, or even someone saying our name [17]. This easy awakening makes evolutionary sense, as our ancestors needed to remain somewhat alert to potential dangers even while beginning to rest.

One of the most fascinating phenomena of N1 sleep is the hypnic jerk—that sudden, startling sensation of falling that many people experience just as they're drifting off [18]. These involuntary muscle twitches, technically called hypnic myoclonia, can feel dramatic enough to jolt us back to wakefulness. While scientists haven't pinpointed the exact cause, these jerks might represent an ancient reflex from our evolutionary past, possibly reflecting an ancient reflex from our evolutionary past, though its precise origin remains debated. They occur as our muscles begin to relax, sometimes triggering a brief protective reflex.

During N1 sleep, our thoughts begin to take on dream-like qualities [19]. If awakened during this stage, people often report experiencing fragmentary visual images or brief, dream-like thoughts. These aren't the elaborate dreams that occur during deeper sleep stages, but rather fleeting snippets that hover between conscious thought and true dreams. Because N1 is so light, people awakened from it usually feel alert and may even question whether they were asleep (Fig. 5.4).

This initial sleep stage also brings physical changes. Our eye movements slow into a gentle rolling pattern, distinct from the rapid movements of wakefulness and those seen later in REM sleep. Our muscle tone starts to decrease, but remains higher than in deeper stages of sleep like N3 or REM. Even our perception of the environment begins to fade, though we remain more aware than in later sleep stages.

Understanding N1 sleep helps explain several common experiences, like why we might deny having dozed off during a boring meeting or while watching television, even though others saw us nodding off. During these brief dips into N1 sleep, we maintain enough awareness that we might not realize we've briefly crossed the threshold into sleep. While meditation might feel similar to this drowsy state, it's actually quite different. During meditation, you remain fully conscious and aware, maintaining what scientists call a "relaxed alertness." Your brain produces alpha and theta waves similar to those seen in early N1 sleep, but unlike sleep, you maintain executive control of your attention. This is why experienced meditators can sit for hours in deep meditation without falling asleep—they're accessing a unique state of consciousness that's neither sleep nor typical wakefulness. The confusion often arises because both states involve reduced physical movement and slower breathing patterns, but while sleep progressively disconnects you from your environment, meditation actually enhances your moment-to-moment awareness of both internal and external experiences.

For most people, N1 serves as a short but necessary transition into deeper sleep stages. However, some individuals with sleep disorders might spend a disproportionate amount of time in light sleep, preventing them from getting the restorative benefits of deeper sleep. This observation has important implications for sleep disorders and their treatment, as helping patients move more efficiently through N1 into deeper sleep stages can significantly improve their sleep quality.

5.1.3.2 Stage N2 Sleep: When Sleep Deepens

After drifting through the light sleep of stage N1, we enter Stage N2, the most prevalent stage of sleep that typically occupies nearly half of our total sleep time [17]. During this stage, our sleep becomes more established, though not yet in our

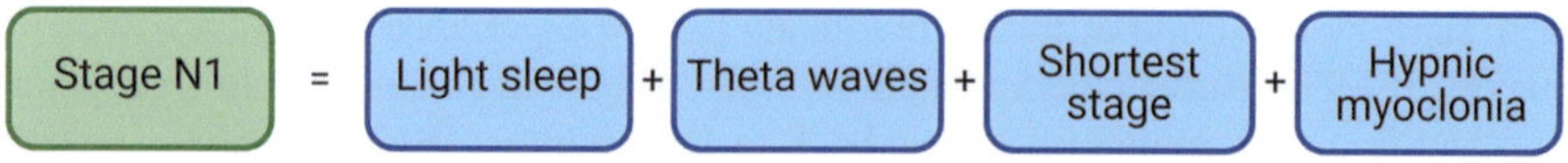

Fig. 5.4 Schematic overview of characteristics of N1 sleep stage. ("Image generated by ChatGPT (OpenAI), 2025. Used with permission")

deepest sleep state. Think of N2 as the middle ground between light and deep sleep, where many processes begin to unfold.

During N2 sleep, our brain produces two distinctive EEG patterns that sleep scientists find particularly intriguing: sleep spindles and K-complexes [17]. Sleep spindles appear as brief bursts of rapid electrical activity, like short sprints of brain waves lasting up to 2 s. These spindles serve as a hallmark of memory consolidation during sleep. These bursts of brain activity support the transfer of information from short-term to long-term memory, helping solidify what we've learned during the day. Research shows that people who generate more sleep spindles often perform better on memory tests the next day [20].

K-complexes, the other hallmark of N2 sleep, appear as dramatic spikes in brain activity—large waves that stand out prominently in sleep recordings [17]. These waves are thought to serve a protective gating function, helping to suppress disruptions that might wake us. When a noise occurs during sleep, a K-complex may be triggered in response. These waveforms help suppress unnecessary brain activity, protecting sleep from mild disruptions. However, if the noise is perceived as potentially important or threatening, the brain may shift toward wakefulness—suggesting K-complexes play a role in both preserving sleep and monitoring the environment. This dual role reflects the brain's remarkable ability to protect both our sleep and our safety (Fig. 5.5).

During N2 sleep, our body continues its transition into deeper sleep [17]. Our heart rate slows further, and our body temperature drops slightly. Eye movements, which might still occur occasionally during N1 sleep, now become rare. Our muscles relax more deeply, though not yet to the level of complete relaxation we'll see in deeper sleep stages.

The prominence of N2 sleep—occupying about 45% of our total sleep time—suggests its vital importance. Beyond memory consolidation, this stage appears crucial for both neural maintenance and physiological recovery. Some scientists believe that the regular rhythms of sleep spindles might help maintain and strengthen neural connections, like a maintenance crew testing and reinforcing electrical circuits while the main power is turned down.

Sleep research into N2 has revealed practical implications for many aspects of daily life. For instance, the relationship between sleep spindles and memory helps explain why a good night's sleep can improve learning and problem-solving abilities. Students studying for exams or professionals learning new skills benefit particularly from getting adequate sleep, as the spindles during N2 help facilitate the transfer of this new knowledge into long-term memory. This stage also helps explain why some people can sleep through minor disturbances while others wake easily. The effectiveness of K-complexes in suppressing arousal varies among individuals,

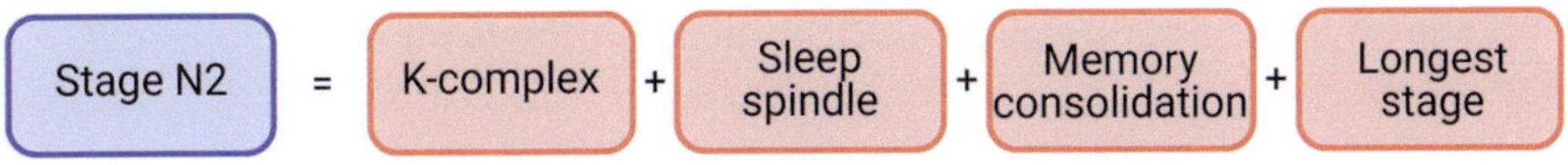

Fig. 5.5 Schematic overview of characteristics of N2 sleep stage. ("Image generated by ChatGPT (OpenAI), 2025. Used with permission")

which might partially explain why some people describe themselves as "light" or "heavy" sleepers, though several other factors play a role here. These findings have informed practical strategies for improving sleep in noisy environments, such as using consistent background noise (white or pink noise) to mask sudden disturbances that might trigger arousal.

5.1.3.3 Stage N3: The Depths of Deep Sleep

When we enter Stage N3 sleep, we reach our deepest, most restorative form of non-REM sleep [17]. Taking up about 25% of our total sleep time, this stage represents what many people refer to as deep sleep. During N3, the brain produces powerful, slow delta waves that dominate the brain's electrical activity, reflecting a deep state of neural synchronization. These waves, much slower and larger than those seen in lighter sleep stages, reflect a level of sleep so deep that waking someone during this stage can leave them feeling groggy, dazed and disoriented for several minutes—a state sleep scientists call "sleep inertia" [21].

During N3 sleep, the brain and body engage in crucial maintenance and restoration work [17]. Like a city's maintenance crew that becomes most active when the streets are empty, the brain activates its remarkable cleaning system during this deep sleep stage. This system, called the glymphatic system, works like the brain's dedicated waste management service. Cerebrospinal fluid flows through the brain's tissues efficiently during deep sleep, thanks to a temporary increase in the space between brain cells, which allows the fluid to circulate more freely and wash away accumulated waste products and toxins that build up during wakefulness.

The importance of this cleaning process becomes clear when we consider its role in brain health. Recent research has revealed that poor sleep can interfere with the glymphatic system's function, potentially leading to the accumulation of proteins associated with neurodegenerative conditions like Alzheimer's disease [22]. When we don't get enough deep sleep, these waste products, including beta-amyloid proteins, can build up over time, potentially contributing to cognitive decline and increased disease risk (Fig. 5.6).

N3 sleep also plays a vital role in memory processing and physical restoration. During this stage, the brain consolidates and integrates new information learned during the day, particularly factual knowledge (declarative memory) and procedural memories, such as learning new physical skills. Growth hormone secretion peaks during N3 sleep, promoting tissue repair and cellular regeneration throughout the body. This explains why deep sleep proves especially important for physical recovery after injury or intense exercise.

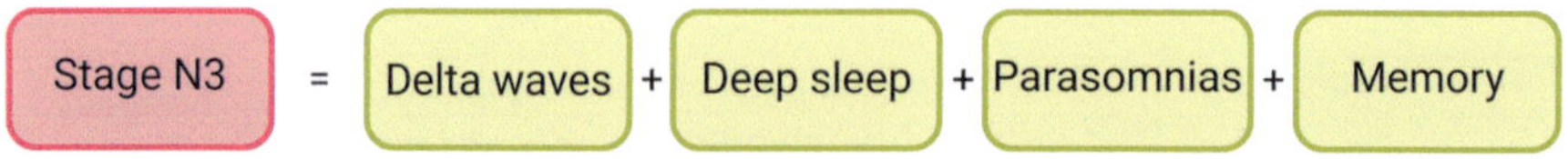

Fig. 5.6 Schematic overview of characteristics of N3 sleep stage. ("Image generated by ChatGPT (OpenAI), 2025. Used with permission")

Interestingly, this stage of sleep can sometimes produce unusual behaviors known as parasomnias [23]. Sleepwalking, sleep talking, and night terrors typically occur during N3 sleep, when the brain exists in a hybrid state—partially asleep and partially awake—allowing complex behaviors to emerge without full consciousness. During these episodes, parts of the brain remain in deep sleep while others become partially activated, leading to complex behaviors that the person typically won't remember the next day. Historically, sleep scientists divided deep sleep into stages N3 and N4 based on the proportion of delta waves present. However, current classification systems generally combine these into a single stage N3, recognizing that they represent a continuous spectrum of deep sleep rather than distinctly different states. This simplified classification better reflects our understanding of sleep's natural progression.

The amount of N3 sleep we get changes throughout our lives. Young children spend more time in this deep sleep stage, which supports their rapid growth and development [17]. In adolescence, N3 sleep remains important for brain maturation, but its proportion begins to decline gradually from childhood onward. As we age, we typically experience less N3 sleep, which may partially explain why older adults often report feeling less refreshed after sleep. This reduction in deep sleep might also contribute to the increased risk of cognitive decline with aging, given N3's crucial role in brain maintenance and memory consolidation.

Deep sleep plays a vital role in our health, and several factors can help us get more of this restorative stage. Regular exercise, particularly earlier in the day, can help us sleep better, including potentially getting more deep sleep. Maintaining a consistent sleep schedule also helps ensure we spend adequate time in this restorative stage. Additionally, avoiding alcohol before bedtime proves important, as alcohol disrupts sleep architecture—reducing deep sleep and increasing nighttime awakenings—even though it may initially promote sleep onset.

5.1.3.4 REM Sleep: The Dream Stage

REM (Rapid Eye Movement) sleep represents one of sleep's most fascinating stages—a period when our brain becomes highly active while our body remains largely paralyzed [17]. Taking up about 25% of our total sleep time, REM sleep typically occurs more frequently in the latter part of the night, which explains why we often remember dreams when waking naturally in the morning. During this stage, our brain activity patterns closely resemble those of wakefulness, leading scientists to call it "paradoxical sleep"—we're deeply asleep, yet our brains are buzzing with activity.

During REM sleep, our body undergoes remarkable changes. While most of our voluntary muscles become temporarily paralyzed (a state called muscle atonia), certain critical muscles remain active—those controlling our eyes, heart, and breathing. Our eyes move back and forth rapidly beneath closed lids, giving this stage its name: Rapid Eye Movement sleep. Our breathing becomes irregular, our heart rate fluctuates, and blood pressure rises as our sympathetic nervous system—normally associated with "fight or flight" responses—becomes more active.

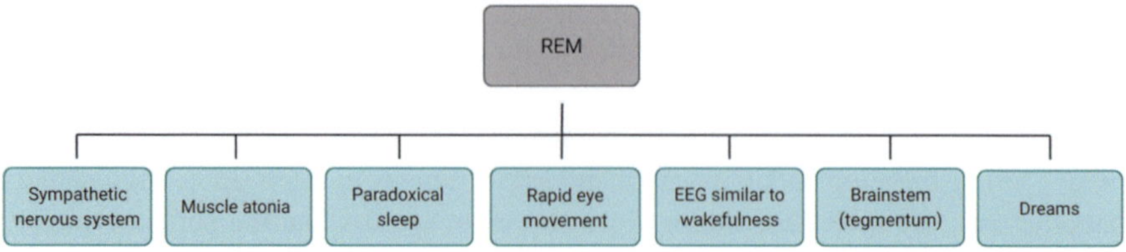

Fig. 5.7 Schematic overview of characteristics of REM sleep stage. ("Image generated by ChatGPT (OpenAI), 2025. Used with permission")

The paralysis of our voluntary muscles during REM sleep serves a crucial protective function. In the 1960s, French scientist Michel Jouvet conducted groundbreaking research showing that damage to specific areas in the brainstem could eliminate this muscle paralysis, causing animals to physically act out their dreams [24]. Jouvet's discovery not only confirmed that REM paralysis is actively regulated by the brainstem, but laid the groundwork for understanding REM sleep behavior disorder (RBD) in humans—a condition where the normal muscle paralysis fails during sleep, allowing people to physically act out their dreams, sometimes with dangerous consequences [25] (Fig. 5.7).

REM sleep plays a vital role in brain function, particularly in memory and learning [17]. While all sleep stages contribute to memory processing, REM sleep appears especially important for emotional memories and complex learning tasks. During REM sleep, the brain might be rehearsing and strengthening neural pathways related to newly learned skills or processing emotional experiences from the day. This explains why sleep often improves both emotional stability and problem-solving abilities. The amount of REM sleep we experience changes dramatically throughout our lives. Newborns spend up to 50% of their sleep time in REM sleep, suggesting its crucial role in early brain development. This proportion declines rapidly over the first year of life and gradually decreases as we age, with older adults typically experiencing less REM sleep than younger people. This reduction might contribute to changes in memory and emotional processing that often occur with aging.

The biology underlying REM sleep involves precise interactions between different brain regions and chemical messengers. The control center for REM sleep lies in the brainstem, specifically in an area called the pons [26]. Here, the neurotransmitter acetylcholine activates REM sleep, while serotonin and other neurotransmitters help modulate its timing and transitions. This delicate chemical balance explains why certain medications that affect these neurotransmitters (e.g., antidepressants) can significantly alter REM sleep, often reducing its duration and vivid dreaming.

Dreaming, while most vivid during REM sleep, can occur throughout all stages of sleep. Although dreams in lighter sleep stages are often less detailed, REM sleep dreams stand out with their rich, complex narratives and heightened emotional intensity. This suggests that REM sleep may play a crucial role in processing our daily emotional experiences, regulating mood, and integrating new information with our existing memories, ultimately contributing to both cognitive function and overall emotional well-being.

The discovery that most mammals and birds experience REM sleep, while reptiles do not, suggests this sleep stage evolved later in vertebrate evolution—likely alongside the emergence of warm-blooded animals with more complex brains. This finding has led scientists to speculate about REM sleep's role in the development of complex cognitive abilities in warm-blooded animals. The fact that animals show signs of dreaming—from twitching whiskers in cats to wing movements in birds—suggests that dream experiences might be more widespread in the animal kingdom than previously thought.

5.1.4 Dreams and Brain Activity

Dreams are among the most intriguing features of sleep. During both REM and non-REM sleep, specific brain regions become active in patterns that create our dream experiences. When we study the sleeping brain, we find that the posterior regions, particularly areas involved in visual processing, show significant activity during dreams. This activity creates vivid visual experiences that can feel as real as waking life, even though our eyes remain closed and our brain receives no input from the outside world.

Different sleep stages produce different types of dreams [19]. During non-REM sleep, especially early in the night, dreams tend to reflect daily activities and recent memories. These dreams usually follow more logical patterns—you might dream about finishing a work project or having a conversation similar to one from earlier that day. In REM sleep, dreams often become surreal, emotionally charged, and less bound by logic, often featuring unusual scenarios. This difference occurs because during REM sleep, brain areas involved in emotion and memory (like the amygdala and hippocampus) become active while regions that handle logical thinking show reduced activity.

Brain imaging studies show that dreams involve many sensory areas working together, much like during wakefulness [27]. While almost all dreams include visual elements, many also contain sounds, and some include sensations of touch, taste, or smell. The brain creates all these sensory experiences internally, without any actual sensory input from the environment. This ability demonstrates how our brain can construct complete multisensory experiences using only its internal resources.

Scientists once thought dreaming occurred only during REM sleep, but research has revealed this isn't true. Dreams can emerge whenever certain patterns of brain activity occur, regardless of sleep stage. Studies show that when awakened from non-REM sleep, about 70% of people can report some form of dream experience, though these dreams often differ from REM dreams in their content and complexity [19]. On the other hand, most dreams fade quickly from memory due to them being stored in short-term memory which retains information for about 30 seconds. Additionally, We're most likely to remember dreams if we wake directly from REM sleep—if we transition to another sleep stage first, that dream experience is less likely to get encoded into long-term memory [28]. This explains why even vivid dreams can slip away within minutes of waking unless immediately recorded.

The emotional content of dreams deserves special attention. During REM sleep, the emotional centers of the brain become highly active while areas that normally help control emotions show decreased activity [29]. This explains why dreams can involve such powerful feelings and why frightening dreams often feel particularly intense. The brain processes emotional experiences during dreams differently than during wakefulness, potentially helping us integrate and make sense of emotional events from our daily lives.

Studying lucid dreams—where people become aware they're dreaming while remaining asleep—has provided valuable insights into how dreams work [30]. During lucid dreams, brain areas associated with self-awareness, particularly in the prefrontal cortex, show increased activity. Some practiced lucid dreamers can even perform specific tasks during their dreams and communicate with researchers using pre-arranged eye movement signals, allowing scientists to study dreams while they're happening.

Dreams also reveal interesting aspects of how our brains process experience and memory. People who are blind from birth can still experience visual dreams, creating mental images based on how they understand objects through their other senses [31]. Similarly, people who have never walked due to congenital paralysis can dream of walking too. These findings suggest that our brains maintain certain fundamental programs and capabilities even without direct experience.

Recent research using advanced brain imaging continues uncovering new details about how dreams form. When someone dreams about seeing faces, the same brain areas activate as when seeing faces while awake [32]. When dreaming about movement, motor planning regions become active [33]. However, one key difference exists—the prefrontal cortex, which helps us think logically while awake, shows reduced activity during most dreams [34]. This explains why we accept unusual or impossible events in dreams without questioning them—our brain's logical analysis system operates differently during sleep.

During sleep, the brain appears to use dreams as part of its process for strengthening important memories and discarding less relevant information. This might explain why dreams often incorporate elements from recent experiences but combine them in new and sometimes unusual ways. The sleeping brain actively processes and reorganizes information, with dreams potentially reflecting this important memory consolidation work. However, while fascinating, the meaning of dreams still has many unanswered questions.

5.1.5 Sleep Versus Anesthesia: Two Different Paths to Altered Consciousness

While sleep and general anesthesia might seem similar on the surface—both involving a loss of consciousness—they represent fundamentally different brain states. General anesthesia combines several distinct elements: unconsciousness, analgesia (prevention of pain), muscle paralysis, and amnesia ("memory blockade") [35]. Each of these components differs from sleep in important ways. For example, sleeping people can still feel pain, process memories, and maintain muscle tone (except during REM sleep when temporary paralysis occurs), whereas general anesthesia deliberately blocks all these functions. Even unconsciousness differs—sleep allows for arousal in response to important stimuli, while anesthetic unconsciousness deliberately prevents any such awareness.

Anesthesia creates a rapid, complete shutdown of consciousness through powerful drugs (e.g., propofol) that target specific brain systems. These medications primarily enhance the effects of GABA, the brain's main inhibitory neurotransmitter [36], rapidly dampening activity across widespread brain areas. This contrasts markedly with sleep's gradual progression, where consciousness dims as different brain areas transition into sleep patterns at varying rates. The transition to sleep involves complex interactions between multiple neurotransmitter systems—not just GABA, but also serotonin, norepinephrine, and acetylcholine [37].

The brain behaves quite differently during sleep compared to anesthesia. During natural sleep, brain activity follows complex, coordinated patterns that evolve throughout the night, with distinct signatures across sleep stages—from the synchronized slow waves of deep sleep to the active patterns of REM sleep. In contrast, anesthesia typically suppresses brain activity more uniformly. Some EEG patterns under anesthesia may superficially resemble those seen in sleep, but the underlying neurobiological mechanisms and the functional outcomes differ substantially. Sleep is a dynamic process of restoration and reorganization, whereas anesthesia creates a controlled state of unconsciousness designed solely for procedural safety.

These differences extend to how the brain processes information. In natural sleep, the brain remains responsive to important signals from the body and environment so that we can awaken quickly if needed. Under anesthesia, this responsiveness largely disappears. Similarly, while dreaming represents a form of consciousness during sleep, anesthesia typically blocks all conscious experience. The thalamus—a key relay station for sensory information—illustrates these differences: during sleep, it filters incoming signals yet retains some processing capacity, while under anesthesia, thalamic activity drops significantly, effectively blocking most sensory processing [38].

The recovery process also differs notably between sleep and anesthesia. Waking from natural sleep generally occurs smoothly, with the brain's systems reactivating in a coordinated manner, delivering the restorative benefits essential for cognitive and emotional health. In contrast, recovery from anesthesia can be more complex, as the brain must clear the anesthetic drugs while reestablishing normal patterns of activity. This highlights how sleep represents a natural, restorative biological rhythm, whereas anesthesia is an artificially induced state essential for surgical procedures, but lacking the recuperative benefits of sleep.

References

1. Borbély A. The two-process model of sleep regulation: beginnings and outlook. J Sleep Res. 2022;31(4):e13598.
2. Peng W, Wu Z, Song K, Zhang S, Li Y, Xu M. Regulation of sleep homeostasis mediator adenosine by basal forebrain glutamatergic neurons. Science. 2020;369(6508):eabb0556.

3. Li SB, de Lecea L. The hypocretin (orexin) system: from a neural circuitry perspective. Neuropharmacology. 2020;167:107993.
4. Szabo ST, Thorpy MJ, Mayer G, Peever JH, Kilduff TS. Neurobiological and immunogenetic aspects of narcolepsy: implications for pharmacotherapy. Sleep Med Rev. 2019;43:23–36.
5. Morairty S, Rainnie D, McCarley R, Greene R. Disinhibition of ventrolateral preoptic area sleep-active neurons by adenosine: a new mechanism for sleep promotion. Neuroscience. 2004;123(2):451–7.
6. Arguinchona JH, Tadi P. Neuroanatomy, reticular activating system. [Updated 2023 Jul 24]. In: StatPearls [Internet]. Treasure Island (FL): StatPearls Publishing; 2025. Available from: https://www.ncbi.nlm.nih.gov/books/NBK549835/
7. Slater C, Liu Y, Weiss E, Yu K, Wang Q. The neuromodulatory role of the noradrenergic and cholinergic systems and their interplay in cognitive functions: a focused review. Brain Sci. 2022;12(7):890.
8. Vellei M, Chinazzo G, Zitting KM, Hubbard J. Human thermal perception and time of day: a review. Temperature (Austin). 2021;8(4):320–41.
9. Duffy JF, Zeitzer JM, Rimmer DW, Klerman EB, Dijk DJ, Czeisler CA. Peak of circadian melatonin rhythm occurs later within the sleep of older subjects. Am J Physiol Endocrinol Metab. 2002;282(2):E297–303.
10. Maeda T, Koga H, Nonaka T, Higuchi S. Effects of bathing-induced changes in body temperature on sleep. J Physiol Anthropol. 2023;42(1):20.
11. Stutz J, Eiholzer R, Spengler CM. Effects of evening exercise on sleep in healthy participants: a systematic review and meta-analysis. Sports Med. 2019;49(2):269–87.
12. American Academy of Sleep Medicine. How to sleep better [Internet]. Darien (IL): AASM; 2024. Available from: https://aasm.org/resources/pdf/products/howtosleepbetter_web.pdf
13. Cerri M, Luppi M, Tupone D, Zamboni G, Amici R. REM sleep and Endothermy: potential sites and mechanism of a reciprocal interference. Front Physiol. 2017;8:624.
14. Nayak CS, Anilkumar AC. EEG normal sleep. [Updated 2023 May 23]. In: StatPearls [Internet]. Treasure Island (FL): StatPearls Publishing; 2025. Available from: https://www.ncbi.nlm.nih.gov/books/NBK537023/
15. Fink AM, Bronas UG, Calik MW. Autonomic regulation during sleep and wakefulness: a review with implications for defining the pathophysiology of neurological disorders. Clin Auton Res. 2018;28(6):509–18.
16. Tudor M, Tudor L, Tudor KI. Hans Berger (1873-1941) – povijest elektroencefalografije [Hans Berger (1873-1941) – the history of electroencephalography]. Acta Med Croatica. 2005;59(4):307–13.
17. Patel AK, Reddy V, Shumway KR, et al. Physiology, sleep stages. [Updated 2024 Jan 26]. In: StatPearls [Internet]. Treasure Island (FL): StatPearls Publishing; 2025. Available from: https://www.ncbi.nlm.nih.gov/books/NBK526132/
18. Kumar R, Ali SN, Saha S, Bhattacharjee S. SSRI induced hypnic jerks: a case series. Indian J Psychiatry. 2023;65(7):785–8.
19. Martin JM, Andriano DW, Mota NB, Mota-Rolim SA, Araújo JF, Solms M, Ribeiro S. Structural differences between REM and non-REM dream reports assessed by graph analysis. PLoS One. 2020;15(7):e0228903.
20. Lustenberger C, Wehrle F, Tüshaus L, Achermann P, Huber R. The multidimensional aspects of sleep spindles and their relationship to word-pair memory consolidation. Sleep. 2015;38(7):1093–103.
21. Hilditch CJ, McHill AW. Sleep inertia: current insights. Nat Sci Sleep. 2019;11:155–65.
22. Chong PLH, Garic D, Shen MD, Lundgaard I, Schwichtenberg AJ. Sleep, cerebrospinal fluid, and the glymphatic system: a systematic review. Sleep Med Rev. 2022 Feb;61:101572.
23. Ariba KA, Tadi P. Parasomnias. [Updated 2023 Jul 17]. In: StatPearls [Internet]. Treasure Island (FL): StatPearls Publishing; 2025. Available from: https://www.ncbi.nlm.nih.gov/books/NBK560524/
24. Arnulf I, Buda C, Sastre JP. Michel Jouvet: an explorer of dreams and a great storyteller. Sleep Med. 2018;49:4–9.

25. Khawaja I, Spurling BC, Singh S. REM sleep behavior disorder. [Updated 2023 Apr 24]. In: StatPearls [Internet]. Treasure Island (FL): StatPearls Publishing; 2025. Available from: https://www.ncbi.nlm.nih.gov/books/NBK534239/
26. Luppi PH, Clement O, Sapin E, Peyron C, Gervasoni D, Léger L, Fort P. Brainstem mechanisms of paradoxical (REM) sleep generation. Pflugers Arch. 2012;463(1):43–52.
27. Nir Y, Tononi G. Dreaming and the brain: from phenomenology to neurophysiology. Trends Cogn Sci. 2010;14(2):88–100.
28. Pappas S. Why do we forget so many of our dreams? Scientific American [Internet]. 2023. Available from: https://www.scientificamerican.com/article/why-do-we-forget-so-many-of-our-dreams
29. Goldstein AN, Walker MP. The role of sleep in emotional brain function. Annu Rev Clin Psychol. 2014;10:679–708.
30. Baird B, Mota-Rolim SA, Dresler M. The cognitive neuroscience of lucid dreaming. Neurosci Biobehav Rev. 2019;100:305–23.
31. Siclari F, Valli K, Arnulf I. Dreams and nightmares in healthy adults and in patients with sleep and neurological disorders. Lancet Neurol. 2020;19(10):849–59.
32. Carr M, Haar A, Amores J, Lopes P, Bernal G, Vega T, Rosello O, Jain A, Maes P. Dream engineering: simulating worlds through sensory stimulation. Conscious Cogn. 2020;83:102955.
33. De Carli F, Proserpio P, Morrone E, Sartori I, Ferrara M, Gibbs SA, De Gennaro L, Lo Russo G, Nobili L. Activation of the motor cortex during phasic rapid eye movement sleep. Ann Neurol. 2016;79(2):326–30.
34. Scarpelli S, Alfonsi V, Gorgoni M, Giannini AM, De Gennaro L. Investigation on neurobiological mechanisms of dreaming in the new decade. Brain Sci. 2021;11(2):220.
35. Brown EN, Pavone KJ, Naranjo M. Multimodal general anesthesia: theory and practice. Anesth Analg. 2018;127(5):1246–58.
36. Brohan J, Goudra BG. The role of GABA receptor agonists in anesthesia and sedation. CNS Drugs. 2017;31(10):845–56.
37. Siegel JM. The neurotransmitters of sleep. J Clin Psychiatry. 2004;65(Suppl 16):4–7.
38. Kantonen O, Laaksonen L, Alkire M, Scheinin A, Långsjö J, Kallionpää RE, Kaisti K, Radek L, Johansson J, Laitio T, Maksimow A, Scheinin J, Nyman M, Scheinin M, Solin O, Vahlberg T, Revonsuo A, Valli K, Scheinin H. Decreased thalamic activity is a correlate for disconnectedness during anesthesia with propofol, dexmedetomidine and sevoflurane but not S-ketamine. J Neurosci. 2023;43(26):4884–95.

Nutrition and Sleep: Dietary Influences on Rest

6

6.1 Food, Drinks, and Sleep: How Diet Affects Our Rest

6.1.1 Caffeine and the Sleep-Wake Cycle

We touched upon caffeine's effect on sleep in the previous sections, but it's worth expanding the conversation as coffee is the most widely consumed psychoactive substance, with an estimated 2.25 billion cups consumed daily worldwide [1]. From ancient trading routes to modern coffee shop culture, this beverage has shaped human society for centuries. While coffee helps millions and millions of people feel alert and focused, its relationship with sleep involves complex biological mechanisms that affect everyone differently.

At the molecular level, caffeine works by interfering with one of sleep's fundamental mechanisms. Earlier, we discussed adenosine, the molecule that accumulates during wakefulness to create sleep pressure. Caffeine's primary action involves blocking adenosine receptors in the brain, particularly the A1 and A2A receptor subtypes [2]. When caffeine molecules attach to these receptors, they prevent adenosine from delivering its sleep-promoting signal. This blockade doesn't eliminate adenosine—the molecule continues to build up—but temporarily prevents the brain from sensing its effects.

The duration of caffeine's effects varies remarkably among individuals. In most healthy adults, it takes about 5 h for the body to eliminate half of the consumed caffeine, a measure known as the "half-life" [3]. However, this timeframe can range from 1.5 to 9.5 h depending on several factors [3]. Genetics play a crucial role—some people carry certain variants of the CYP1A2 gene that affect how quickly their liver metabolizes caffeine [4]. This gene produces the primary enzyme responsible for breaking down caffeine, and genetic variations can make some people either "fast" or "slow" metabolizers. For slow metabolizers, a 2 PM coffee might still affect their sleep at 10 PM, as a substantial amount of caffeine remains active in their bloodstream and brain due to their reduced rate of caffeine breakdown and elimination. In contrast, fast metabolizers might be able to

A. Juginović, *Sleep Science Made Simple*,
https://doi.org/10.1007/978-3-031-92060-8_6

metabolize and eliminate the same amount of caffeine in just a few hours with minimal impact on their sleep. Approximately 12% of the population are slow metabolizers due to specific CYP1A2 variants, while others may process caffeine at average speed or quickly [5]. Additional genes, including ADORA2A, influence how sensitive people are to caffeine's effects on sleep, explaining why some individuals can drink coffee before bed while others experience insomnia from a morning cup [6]. Other factors affecting caffeine metabolism include liver function, hormone levels, medication use, and even smoking status, with smokers processing caffeine about twice as fast as non-smokers [7]. Women taking oral contraceptives typically metabolize caffeine more slowly, as estrogen compounds compete for the same metabolic pathways [8]. Similarly, pregnancy can significantly slow caffeine metabolism, with the half-life potentially extending to 15 h during the third trimester [9].

The impact of caffeine on sleep architecture—the distinct stages of sleep—proves particularly interesting. While caffeine primarily affects sleep onset (how quickly we fall asleep), it also reduces the amount of deep sleep, technically called slow-wave sleep [10]. This deep sleep plays crucial roles in physical restoration and memory consolidation, making its reduction potentially significant for overall health. Caffeine can also increase the number of brief micro-awakenings during the night, even if we don't remember them the next day [11].

Age significantly influences caffeine sensitivity. As we age, our ability to metabolize caffeine often slows, and our sleep becomes naturally lighter and more fragmented [12]. For older adults, even moderate caffeine consumption—a standard cup of coffee containing 90-100 mg—can significantly impact sleep quality when consumed in the afternoon or evening [13]. This age-related sensitivity partly explains why many older adults find they need to reduce their caffeine intake or restrict it to morning hours.

Individual differences in caffeine response extend beyond genetics and age. Regular coffee drinkers often develop some tolerance to caffeine's effects, though this tolerance rarely becomes complete. Time of consumption matters significantly—morning caffeine generally affects sleep less than afternoon or evening consumption. Even factors like body weight, food consumption, and overall health status can influence how caffeine affects an individual's sleep.

For optimal sleep, understanding your personal caffeine sensitivity becomes really important. This involves paying attention to how different amounts and timing of caffeine consumption affect your sleep quality. Keep track of when you consume caffeine-containing beverages and foods (including green/black tea, chocolate, and some soft drinks) and how they relate to your sleep patterns. Note that some people are sensitive not just to caffeine's direct effects but also to its indirect impacts on anxiety or heart rate, both of which can disrupt sleep.

The relationship between caffeine and sleep represents a balance between its benefits for daytime alertness and its potential to disrupt rest. While current research suggests that moderate coffee consumption—up to 200–300 mg of caffeine daily for most healthy adults—generally proves safe, timing this consumption appropriately becomes key for maintaining healthy sleep patterns [14].

6.1.2 What We Eat Affects How We Sleep

Why do some meals leave you drowsy, while others make it harder to fall asleep? The relationship between food and sleep operates through multiple pathways, with both meal timing and food choices significantly affecting sleep quality. Because your circadian rhythm regulates both metabolism and sleep, when you eat can directly impact how well you sleep. Large meals consumed close to bedtime can disrupt sleep in several ways: they increase your body temperature when it should be cooling down for sleep, boost your metabolism when it should be slowing, and keep your digestive system active when it should be winding down [15, 16]. Carbohydrates and proteins work together in various ways to influence sleep. Proteins provide tryptophan, an amino acid your body uses to produce serotonin and melatonin—key chemicals involved in relaxation and sleep [17]. However, tryptophan needs help getting to your brain, and this is where carbohydrates come in. When you eat carbohydrates, they trigger insulin release, which helps tryptophan cross into the brain more efficiently. This might explain why a small, balanced snack combining complex carbohydrates with protein (like whole grain crackers with cheese) might help you sleep, while a heavy, high-fat meal could disturb it. Research suggests waiting at least 2–3 h after your last substantial meal before going to bed, giving your body time to properly digest before sleep [18].

Certain nutrients play particularly important roles in sleep regulation. Magnesium, found abundantly in leafy greens, nuts, and whole grains, helps activate the parasympathetic nervous system responsible for relaxation and supports GABA production—a neurotransmitter essential for sleep [19, 20]. Foods rich in B vitamins, particularly B6, support the production of both serotonin and melatonin [21]. Bananas, for instance, provide both magnesium and B6, potentially explaining their reputation as a bedtime snack [22]. Tryptophan-rich foods such as turkey, eggs, and dairy products may support sleep, though their effectiveness depends largely on when and how they're consumed [18, 23]. The old advice about warm milk before bed may work not just through tryptophan content but also through its calming ritual and the mild warming effect, which may promote body temperature regulation before sleep. We will go into detail about the measurable impact of various supplements on sleep in one of the next chapters.

The glycemic index—how rapidly a food raises blood sugar—also affects how quickly we fall asleep and the quality of our rest. High-glycemic meals (those that cause a rapid spike in blood sugar, such as white rice or potatoes) consumed 4 h before bedtime have been shown to reduce the time needed to fall asleep, potentially by affecting the ratio of tryptophan to other amino acids in the blood [24]. Sugary foods consumed closer to bedtime can trigger blood sugar fluctuations that disrupt sleep continuity. Low-fiber, high-saturated-fat diets correlate with lighter, less restorative sleep and more nighttime arousals, while Mediterranean-style diets rich in fiber, healthy fats, and complex carbohydrates associate with better sleep quality [25].

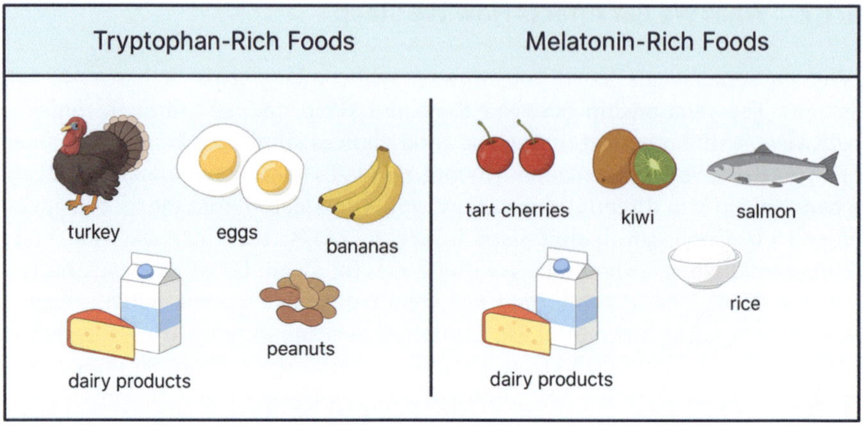

Fig. 6.1 Visual guide to Tryptophan-rich foods and melatonin-rich foods. (''Image generated by ChatGPT (OpenAI), 2025. Used with permission'')

Surprisingly, some foods contain natural sources of melatonin. Tart cherries, particularly Montmorency cherries, contain significant amounts of melatonin and have been shown in clinical studies to improve both sleep onset and duration [26]. Similarly, kiwi fruit consumption 1 h before bedtime improved sleep onset, duration, and efficiency in clinical trials, though the exact mechanism remains unclear—it might involve their high antioxidant content, serotonin levels, or folate content [27]. Fatty fish consumption correlates with better sleep quality, possibly due to their vitamin D and omega-3 content, which help regulate serotonin production [28] (Fig. 6.1).

Fasting and meal timing can also influence our circadian rhythms. Food intake acts as a powerful zeitgeber (time cue) for peripheral clocks, particularly in the liver and digestive system [29]. However, the effects of fasting on sleep are mixed [30].

6.1.3 Alcohol and Sleep: A Deceptive Relationship

Why does that glass of wine help you fall asleep only to wake you up in the middle of the night? While alcohol may seem to help with sleep, its on sleep quality tells a more complicated story. Alcohol acts as a sedative at first, making you feel drowsy and relaxed, but as your body metabolizes it throughout the night, it significantly disrupts your sleep architecture—the natural pattern and structure of your sleep [31].

When you drink alcohol before bed, it initially makes falling asleep easier by increasing a brain chemical called GABA that helps you feel relaxed [32]. But as your body metabolizes the alcohol, it creates what sleep scientists call a "rebound effect" [33]. This typically happens in the second half of the night, when alcohol's sedating effects wear off, often leaving you tossing and turning. This often explains those 3 AM awakenings after evening drinks, even if falling asleep was easy.

Alcohol particularly disrupts REM sleep—the stage where most dreaming occurs and which plays a crucial role in emotional processing and memory consolidation

[34]. Even moderate alcohol intake can suppress REM sleep early in the night. The brain often compensates for this loss by increasing REM sleep later in the night, which fragments sleep and reduces its restorative quality. This REM rebound might explain why people often report vivid or unusual dreams after drinking.

The effects of alcohol on sleep change throughout the night. During the first half of your sleep, when blood alcohol levels are high, you might experience more deep sleep than usual. However, this isn't the good quality deep sleep your body needs. As your liver breaks down the alcohol, sleep becomes increasingly disturbed. This also explains why alcohol leads to more nighttime bathroom visits—by suppressing vasopressin, a hormone that normally helps your body retain water, alcohol increases urine production, leading to more frequent trips to the bathroom during the night.

Individual factors significantly influence how alcohol affects your sleep [34]. Age matters—older adults generally experience more sleep disruption from alcohol than younger people. Your typical drinking patterns play a role too—regular drinkers might not notice these effects as much due to tolerance, though their sleep quality still suffers. Genetics also influence how efficiently you metabolize alcohol—and how much it disrupts your sleep.

For better sleep, one should avoid alcohol for at least 3 h before bedtime. If you do drink in the evening, staying hydrated by drinking water alongside alcohol may help minimize sleep disruption.

6.1.4 Sleep Supplements: What Works and What Doesn't

Can supplements really help you sleep better? While the sleep supplement industry has exploded into a multi-billion dollar market, research reveals a more nuanced picture of what works and what doesn't. From melatonin to magnesium, herbal remedies to amino acids, understanding the science behind these supplements helps you make informed choices about their use.

Melatonin, perhaps the most well-known sleep supplement, works best in specific situations rather than as a general sleep aid. Your body naturally produces this hormone every evening when darkness falls, signaling that it's time to sleep. As a supplement, melatonin is most effective for jet lag, shift work, or circadian rhythm disorders, situations where your internal clock needs resetting, rather than chronic insomnia [35, 36]. However, the correct timing matters more than the dose—taking it approximately 30–60 min before your desired bedtime typically works better than taking it right at bedtime, as it takes around 30–60 min for melatonin to reach its peak levels in your blood [37]. Importantly, more doesn't mean better—most research shows that even smaller doses (0.5–1 mg) work well [37].

Magnesium is a popular sleep aid, and while it may offer some benefit for sleep, the evidence is not particularly strong [38]. This mineral helps "calm" the nervous system and supports the production of brain chemicals that promote relaxation. Many people don't get enough magnesium from their diet, especially as they age [39]. Different forms of magnesium affect the body differently—magnesium glycinate tends to cause less digestive upset than magnesium oxide, for instance.

However, like any supplement, more isn't necessarily better, and high doses can cause digestive issues.

Herbal supplements like valerian root and chamomile have long histories of use for sleep. While research results vary and suggest only modest benefits, these herbs appear to promote relaxation rather than directly inducing sleep [40, 41]. This explains why a cup of chamomile tea might help you unwind but won't knock you out like a sleeping pill. The effects often build over time rather than working immediately, and individual responses can vary significantly.

Some newer supplements show promise but need more research with the current results being mixed. L-theanine, an amino acid found in tea, appears to promote relaxation without drowsiness [42]. Ashwagandha, an herb used in traditional Indian medicine, might help reduce anxiety and improve sleep quality [43]. However, most supplements, including combinations of various supplements, lack the rigorous testing required for medications, making quality and dosing less consistent.

Timing and dosage matter for any supplement, but for most of them the evidence for improving sleep remains limited. Remember that supplements can interact with medications and aren't suitable for everyone—pregnant women, people with certain medical conditions, and those taking other medications should consult healthcare providers before beginning any supplement routine.

References

1. Hou C, Zeng Y, Chen W, Han X, Yang H, Ying Z, Hu Y, Sun Y, Qu Y, Fang F, Song H. Medical conditions associated with coffee consumption: disease-trajectory and comorbidity network analyses of a prospective cohort study in UK biobank. Am J Clin Nutr. 2022;116(3):730–40.
2. Huang ZL, Qu WM, Eguchi N, Chen JF, Schwarzschild MA, Fredholm BB, Urade Y, Hayaishi O. Adenosine A2A, but not A1, receptors mediate the arousal effect of caffeine. Nat Neurosci. 2005;8(7):858–9.
3. Institute of Medicine (US) Committee on Military Nutrition Research. Caffeine for the sustainment of mental task performance: formulations for military operations. Washington National Academies Press (US); 2001, p. 2. Pharmacology of Caffeine. Available from: https://www.ncbi.nlm.nih.gov/books/NBK223808
4. Mahdavi S, Palatini P, El-Sohemy A. CYP1A2 genetic variation, coffee intake, and kidney dysfunction. JAMA Netw Open. 2023;6(1):e2247868.
5. Pittsley RA, Kolomyjec SH. Analysis of the CYP1A2 caffeine metabolism gene in the student population at Lake Superior State University [Preprint]. bioRxiv; 2022. Available from: https://doi.org/10.1101/2022.06.14.496190
6. Landolt HP. "No thanks, coffee keeps me awake": individual caffeine sensitivity depends on ADORA2A genotype. Sleep. 2012;35(7):899–900.
7. Cappelletti S, Piacentino D, Sani G, Aromatario M. Caffeine: cognitive and physical performance enhancer or psychoactive drug? Curr Neuropharmacol. 2015;13(1):71–88. https://doi.org/10.2174/1570159X13666141210215655. Erratum in: Curr Neuropharmacol. 2015;13(4):554. Daria, Piacentino [corrected to Piacentino, Daria]
8. Temple JL, Bernard C, Lipshultz SE, Czachor JD, Westphal JA, Mestre MA. The safety of ingested caffeine: a comprehensive review. Front Psych. 2017;8:80.

9. Lakin H, Sheehan P, Soti V. Maternal caffeine consumption and its impact on the fetus: a review. Cureus. 2023;15(11):e48266.
10. Gardiner C, Weakley J, Burke LM, Roach GD, Sargent C, Maniar N, Townshend A, Halson SL. The effect of caffeine on subsequent sleep: a systematic review and meta-analysis. Sleep Med Rev. 2023;69:101764.
11. Pauchon B, Beauchamps V, Gomez-Mérino D, Erblang M, Drogou C, Beers PV, Guillard M, Quiquempoix M, Léger D, Chennaoui M, Sauvet F. Caffeine intake alters recovery sleep after sleep deprivation. Nutrients. 2024;16:3442.
12. Vestal RE, Norris AH, Tobin JD, Cohen BH, Shock NW, Andres R. Antipyrine metabolism in man: influence of age, alcohol, caffeine, and smoking. Clin Pharmacol Ther. 1975;18(4):425–32.
13. Massey LK. Caffeine and the elderly. Drugs Aging. 1998;13(1):43–50.
14. Rodak K, Kokot I, Kratz EM. Caffeine as a factor influencing the functioning of the human body-friend or foe? Nutrients. 2021;13(9):3088.
15. Driver HS, Shulman I, Baker FC, Buffenstein R. Energy content of the evening meal alters nocturnal body temperature but not sleep. Physiol Behav. 1999;68(1–2):17–23.
16. Crispim CA, Zimberg IZ, dos Reis BG, Diniz RM, Tufik S, de Mello MT. Relationship between food intake and sleep pattern in healthy individuals. J Clin Sleep Med. 2011;7(6):659–64.
17. Paredes SD, Barriga C, Reiter RJ, Rodríguez AB. Assessment of the potential role of tryptophan as the precursor of serotonin and melatonin for the aged sleep-wake cycle and immune function: Streptopelia Risoria as a model. Int J Tryptophan Res. 2009;2:23–36.
18. Chung N, Bin YS, Cistulli PA, Chow CM. Does the proximity of meals to bedtime influence the sleep of young adults? A cross-sectional survey of university students. Int J Environ Res Public Health. 2020;17(8):2677.
19. Gröber U, Schmidt J, Kisters K. Magnesium in prevention and therapy. Nutrients. 2015;7(9):8199–226.
20. Pickering G, Mazur A, Trousselard M, Bienkowski P, Yaltsewa N, Amessou M, Noah L, Pouteau E. Magnesium status and stress: the vicious circle concept revisited. Nutrients. 2020;12(12):3672.
21. Kautz A, Meng Y, Yeh KL, Peck R, Brunner J, Best M, Fernandez ID, Miller RK, Barrett ES, Groth SW, O'Connor TG. Dietary intake of nutrients involved in serotonin and melatonin synthesis and prenatal maternal sleep quality and affective symptoms. J Nutr Metab. 2024;2024:6611169.
22. Falcomer AL, Riquette RFR, de Lima BR, Ginani VC, Zandonadi RP. Health benefits of green banana consumption: a systematic review. Nutrients. 2019;11(6):1222.
23. Zuraikat FM, Wood RA, Barragán R, St-Onge MP. Sleep and diet: mounting evidence of a cyclical relationship. Annu Rev Nutr. 2021;41:309–32.
24. Gangwisch JE, Hale L, St-Onge MP, Choi L, LeBlanc ES, Malaspina D, Opler MG, Shadyab AH, Shikany JM, Snetselaar L, Zaslavsky O, Lane D. High glycemic index and glycemic load diets as risk factors for insomnia: analyses from the Women's Health Initiative. Am J Clin Nutr. 2020;111(2):429–39.
25. Godos J, Ferri R, Lanza G, Caraci F, Vistorte AOR, Yelamos Torres V, Grosso G, Castellano S. Mediterranean diet and sleep features: a systematic review of current evidence. Nutrients. 2024;16(2):282.
26. Howatson G, Bell PG, Tallent J, Middleton B, McHugh MP, Ellis J. Effect of tart cherry juice (Prunus cerasus) on melatonin levels and enhanced sleep quality. Eur J Nutr. 2012;51(8):909–16.
27. Doherty R, Madigan S, Nevill A, Warrington G, Ellis JG. The impact of kiwifruit consumption on the sleep and recovery of elite athletes. Nutrients. 2023;15(10):2274.
28. Del Brutto OH, Mera RM, Ha JE, Gillman J, Zambrano M, Castillo PR. Dietary fish intake and sleep quality: a population-based study. Sleep Med. 2016;17:126–8.
29. Lewis P, Oster H, Korf HW, Foster RG, Erren TC. Food as a circadian time cue – evidence from human studies. Nat Rev Endocrinol. 2020;16(4):213–23.
30. McStay M, Gabel K, Cienfuegos S, Ezpeleta M, Lin S, Varady KA. Intermittent fasting and sleep: a review of human trials. Nutrients. 2021;13(10):3489.

31. Colrain IM, Nicholas CL, Baker FC. Alcohol and the sleeping brain. Handb Clin Neurol. 2014;125:415–31.
32. Lobo IA, Harris RA. GABA(A) receptors and alcohol. Pharmacol Biochem Behav. 2008;90(1):90–4.
33. Roehrs T, Roth T. Sleep, sleepiness, and alcohol use. Alcohol Res Health. 2001;25(2):101–9.
34. Ebrahim IO, Shapiro CM, Williams AJ, Fenwick PB. Alcohol and sleep I: effects on normal sleep. Alcohol Clin Exp Res. 2013;37(4):539–49.
35. Reid KJ, Abbott SM. Jet lag and shift work disorder. Sleep Med Clin. 2015;10(4):523–35.
36. Sateia MJ, Buysse DJ, Krystal AD, Neubauer DN, Heald JL. Clinical practice guideline for the pharmacologic treatment of chronic insomnia in adults: an American Academy of sleep medicine clinical practice guideline. J Clin Sleep Med. 2017;13(2):307–49.
37. Zisapel N. New perspectives on the role of melatonin in human sleep, circadian rhythms and their regulation. Br J Pharmacol. 2018;175(16):3190–9.
38. Arab A, Rafie N, Amani R, Shirani F. The role of magnesium in sleep health: a systematic review of available literature. Biol Trace Elem Res. 2023;201(1):121–8.
39. National Institutes of Health, Office of Dietary Supplements. Magnesium [Internet]. Bethesda (MD): NIH; 2024. Available from: https://ods.od.nih.gov/factsheets/Magnesium-HealthProfessional
40. Bent S, Padula A, Moore D, Patterson M, Mehling W. Valerian for sleep: a systematic review and meta-analysis. Am J Med. 2006;119(12):1005–12.
41. Hieu TH, Dibas M, Surya Dila KA, Sherif NA, Hashmi MU, Mahmoud M, Trang NTT, Abdullah L, Nghia TLB, et al. Therapeutic efficacy and safety of chamomile for state anxiety, generalized anxiety disorder, insomnia, and sleep quality: a systematic review and meta-analysis of randomized trials and quasi-randomized trials. Phytother Res. 2019;33(6):1604–15.
42. Hidese S, Ogawa S, Ota M, Ishida I, Yasukawa Z, Ozeki M, Kunugi H. Effects of L-Theanine administration on stress-related symptoms and cognitive functions in healthy adults: a randomized controlled trial. Nutrients. 2019;11(10):2362.
43. Cheah KL, Norhayati MN, Husniati Yaacob L, Abdul RR. Effect of Ashwagandha (Withania somnifera) extract on sleep: a systematic review and meta-analysis. PLoS One. 2021;16(9):e0257843.

Part II

Sleep: A Foundation of Health and Longevity

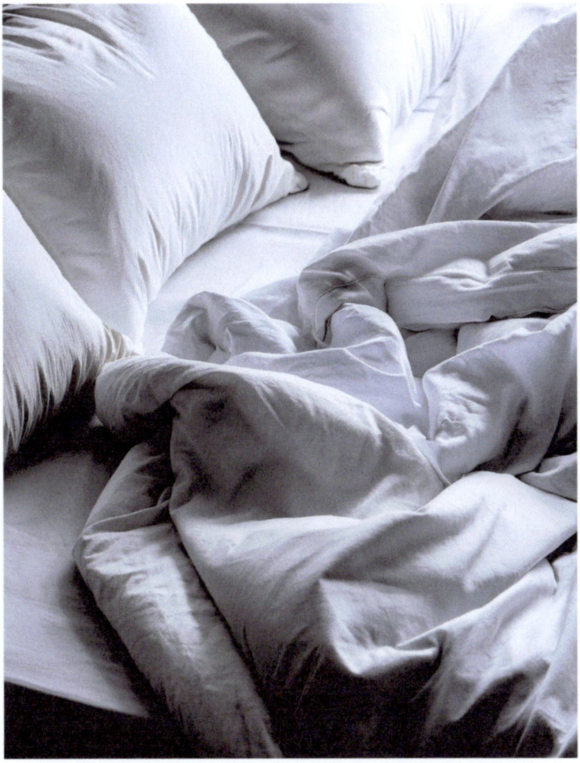

Fig. 1 Transitional 1. (Image generated using the prompt "White bed and pillows; modern style illustration," by Adobe, Adobe Firefly, 2024. (https://firefly.adobe.com/))

Sleep as a Key Pillar for Health Optimization

7

7.1 Beyond Rest: Sleep's Critical Role in Health Optimization

Sleep represents one of our most essential biological processes, far more complex and vital than merely providing rest. During these hours of slumber, our bodies and brains engage in restoration and maintenance processes that affect every aspect of our health. While we might appear still and quiet on the outside, internally the body carries out complex processes of repair, renewal, and optimization. This is why sleep should be considered a whole body process, rather than brain centric.

Each night of sleep triggers comprehensive restoration throughout the body [1]. Muscles repair microscopic damage from daily use, the immune system strengthens its defenses, and hormones regulate everything from growth to appetite. In the brain, sleep enables crucial maintenance operations that we're only beginning to understand. Memory consolidation transforms short-term memories into long-term storage, analyzing and connecting new information with existing knowledge. Through synaptic pruning, the brain refines neural connections, removing unnecessary pathways while strengthening important ones—a process essential for learning and adaptation.

Sleep touches virtually every system of our body [2]. During these crucial hours, the body conducts vital maintenance: the cardiovascular system repairs blood vessels and regulates pressure, while the endocrine system releases growth hormone to regenerate cells and tissues. The immune system synthesizes compounds that combat infection and inflammation, essentially conducting a nightly defense strategy. During sleep, the brain activates the glymphatic system, a cleaning mechanism that flushes out potentially harmful waste that accumulate during wakefulness [3]. This includes beta-amyloid, a protein associated with Alzheimer's disease, highlighting sleep's role in long-term brain health.

The consequences of insufficient sleep ripple throughout the body [4]. Even a single night of poor sleep can affect mood, attention, and decision-making. Chronic sleep deprivation creates more serious disruptions: metabolism becomes impaired,

A. Juginović, *Sleep Science Made Simple*,
https://doi.org/10.1007/978-3-031-92060-8_7

increasing the risk of obesity and diabetes; the immune system weakens, making us more susceptible to infections; blood pressure regulation suffers, raising cardiovascular risks; and cognitive functions decline, affecting everything from reaction time to emotional stability.

Sleep quality proves particularly important for mental health [5]. During sleep, the brain processes emotional experiences, helping maintain psychological well-being. This helps explain why sleep disruption often precedes or worsens mood disorders. The relationship works both ways—poor sleep can contribute to anxiety and depression, while these conditions can make it harder to sleep well.

Perhaps most visibly, sleep transforms our skin [6]. Just one or two nights of missed sleep can dramatically alter our appearance—leading to pale, sallow skin, pronounced dark circles, drooping eyelids, and diminished muscle tone. This occurs because skin repair peaks during slow-wave sleep, when blood flow increases, cortisol drops, and growth hormone surges. Without adequate rest, these regenerative processes get significantly impaired. Yawning, that ubiquitous sign of exhaustion, is itself a peculiar physiological response and we're not sure why it happens [7]. When brain temperature increases, yawning may trigger a cooling mechanism through increased blood flow from jaw movement and heat exchange with cooler ambient air during inhalation. This hypothesis is strengthened by studies showing people yawn significantly more in winter (45%) than in summer (24%), with yawning decreasing when outdoor temperatures exceed body temperature. Researchers identified a "thermal window"—an optimal temperature range for yawning—suggesting this reflex helps maintain ideal brain temperature, another subtle indicator of our body's intricate sleep mechanisms [8].

Understanding sleep's fundamental role in health highlights why protecting sleep should be a priority in our daily lives. Just as we plan our diets and exercise routines, we need to actively manage our sleep habits. This means not only allocating enough time for sleep but also creating conditions that promote quality rest.

The following chapters will explore in detail how sleep affects various aspects of health, from metabolic function to cognitive performance. We'll examine the scientific evidence linking sleep to specific health outcomes and discuss practical strategies for optimizing sleep quality. This knowledge provides the foundation for understanding why good sleep habits represent one of the most significant investments we can make in our long-term health and well-being.

References

1. Irwin MR. Why sleep is important for health: a psychoneuroimmunology perspective. Annu Rev Psychol. 2015;66:143–172. PMID: 25061767.
2. Ramar K, Malhotra RK, Carden KA, Martin JL, Abbasi-Feinberg F, Aurora RN, Kapur VK, Olson EJ, Rosen CL, Rowley JA, Shelgikar AV, Trotti LM. Sleep is essential to health: an American Academy of Sleep Medicine position statement. J Clin Sleep Med. 2021;17(10):2115–2119. PMID: 34170250.
3. Chong PLH, Garic D, Shen MD, Lundgaard I, Schwichtenberg AJ. Sleep, cerebrospinal fluid, and the glymphatic system: a systematic review. Sleep Med Rev. 2022;61:101572. PMID: 34902819.

4. Chattu VK, Manzar MD, Kumary S, Burman D, Spence DW, Pandi-Perumal SR. The global problem of insufficient sleep and its serious public health implications. Healthcare (Basel). 2018;7(1):1. PMID: 30577441.
5. Scott AJ, Webb TL, Martyn-St James M, Rowse G, Weich S. Improving sleep quality leads to better mental health: a meta-analysis of randomised controlled trials. Sleep Med Rev. 2021;60:101556. PMID: 34607184.
6. Oyetakin-White P, Suggs A, Koo B, Matsui. MS, Yarosh D, Cooper KD, Baron ED. Does poor sleep quality affect skin ageing? Clin Exp Dermatol. 2015;40(1):17–22. PMID: 25266053.
7. Giganti F, Zilli I, Aboudan S, Salzarulo P. Sleep, sleepiness and yawning. Front Neurol Neurosci. 2010;28:42–46. PMID: 20357461.
8. Gallup AC, Eldakar OT. Contagious yawning and seasonal climate variation. Front Evol Neurosci. 2011;3:3. PMID: 21960970.

8 Sleep and Cognitive Performance: Learning, Memory, and Mental Clarity

8.1 Sleep's Role in Learning and Cognitive Effects of Poor Sleep

Sleep actively processes our daily experiences, strengthens our memories, and prepares our brains for future learning. This process proves far more complex than simply storing information—it involves sorting, connecting, and refining our experiences and knowledge through neuroplasticity, the brain's ability to physically reshape connections between brain cells to form new neural pathways [1]. The effects of sleep deprivation go beyond learning and memory: even a single night of poor sleep affects our cognitive function, with impacts ranging from basic attention to complex decision-making [1]. These effects translate into real-world consequences, from decreased academic performance to potentially critical errors in high-stakes professions.

To understand how sleep affects memory formation and retention, we first need to examine how our memory systems function and what happens when sleep disrupts these delicate processes. Our memory system operates through three distinct but interconnected components—sensory, short-term, and long-term memory—each playing a vital role in how we process and store information. Sensory memory acts as an initial gateway, capturing the constant stream of information from our environment—the sights, sounds, smells, and tactile sensations. This sensory information remains briefly, lasting only seconds, much like a camera's buffer briefly storing images before processing [2, 3]. From there, important information transfers to short-term memory, primarily processed in the prefrontal cortex, holding about 5–7 items for roughly 15–30 s [2]. This limited capacity explains why you might struggle to remember a phone number if you don't write it down or repeat it immediately. Long-term memory, situated primarily in the temporal lobe, serves as the brain's durable storage system, with the hippocampus acting as a crucial bridge between short-term and long-term memory [4]. Most of this transfer occurs during deep sleep, when the brain experiences its slowest electrical patterns in the form of delta waves [4]. Working memory allows us to actively manipulate information—like

A. Juginović, *Sleep Science Made Simple*,
https://doi.org/10.1007/978-3-031-92060-8_8

solving a math problem or following complex instructions—by drawing on both short-term input and long-term knowledge.

Different sleep stages serve distinct roles in memory processing. During deep sleep, also called slow-wave sleep, the brain transfers information from temporary to long-term storage [4]. This process involves repeated activation of neural circuits, strengthening connections between neurons that represent related pieces of information [5]. During REM sleep, the brain strengthens these stored memories at the cellular level, making them more resistant to forgetting [5]. Stage N2 sleep, characterized by brief bursts of brain activity called sleep spindles, plays a particularly important role in memory transfer. These spindles, which last less than a second, are thought to facilitate the transfer of memories from the hippocampus to the cortex for long-term storage [5]. Scientists can actually observe these spindles using brain monitoring equipment called electroencephalography (EEG), watching as the brain transfers information from temporary to long-term storage [4].

Sleep actively organizes memories, not just storing them [4]. During sleep, the brain sorts through the day's experiences, identifying patterns and making connections with existing knowledge. This process explains why solutions to problems often come to us after a good night's sleep—our brains have been quietly processing and connecting information in new ways. Even a single night of poor sleep can disrupt this process, as demonstrated by research showing that sleeping with lights on impaired both working memory and brain activation patterns [4].

When sleep becomes impaired, whether through insufficient duration or poor quality despite optimal duration, the consequences for learning and memory are significant. The brain's ability to transfer information from short-term to long-term storage becomes compromised, as the crucial processes that occur during different sleep stages—particularly during slow-wave sleep and sleep spindles—are disrupted [5]. This disruption affects not only the consolidation of new memories but also the integration of fresh information with existing knowledge. Sleep-deprived students often struggle to retain new material and recall previously learned concepts, while also experiencing difficulties with basic attention and complex problem-solving tasks. Even a single night of poor sleep can interfere with working memory and cognitive performance, making it harder to learn new material or apply existing knowledge effectively [6]. Additionally, the brain's ability to strengthen motor memories and physical skills becomes compromised, affecting everything from athletic performance to musical practice.

Physical skill learning also depends heavily on sleep and becomes impaired when sleep is inadequate [6]. Whether practicing a sport, learning a musical instrument, or mastering a dance routine, the brain uses sleep to refine and strengthen motor memories. During sleep, the brain replays physical movements learned during the day, strengthening the neural pathways that control these movements. This process, called motor memory consolidation, explains why athletes and musicians often perform better after a good night's sleep [6].

While sleep's effects on memory and learning represent one crucial aspect of brain function, they are part of sleep's broader influence on cognition. The impact of sleep deprivation extends far beyond these fundamental processes, affecting nearly every aspect of how our brains process and respond to information. From basic attention to complex decision-making, understanding how sleep loss impairs cognitive performance reveals why adequate sleep is essential for optimal brain function.

These disruptions to cognitive function manifest through multiple, measurable channels [7]. Brain imaging and performance testing reveal distinct patterns of impairment, with effects that compound over time. These deficits translate into consequential real-world impacts, from calculation errors in financial sectors to critical mistakes in high-stakes medical procedures. The neural mechanisms underlying these effects help explain why sleep plays such a fundamental role in maintaining our cognitive capabilities, beyond its impact on memory and learning.

Sleep deprivation impairs a broad spectrum of cognitive abilities essential for daily functioning [7]. Attention span shortens, making it difficult to focus on tasks or filter out distractions. Processing speed slows, increasing reaction times and reducing efficiency in both simple and complex tasks. Executive functions—including decision-making, planning, and problem-solving—become compromised, leading to poor judgment and increased risk-taking. Working memory capacity diminishes, making it harder to hold and manipulate information in mind. Even basic abilities like language processing and mathematical calculation become less accurate, while higher-order thinking skills like creative problem-solving and cognitive flexibility show marked decline.

These deficits begin at the neural level, where sleep loss produces specific, measurable changes in brain activity. EEG recordings during sleep deprivation show disrupted patterns of neural activity—particularly in the temporal and parietal lobes [8, 9]. These regions, crucial for information processing and integration, show reduced activity after sleep loss. These effects often worsen progressively as sleep debt accumulates, leading to measurable deficits in cognitive testing.

While normal sleep supports optimal cognitive functioning through multiple mechanisms, sleep loss directly impairs these processes. The prefrontal cortex—responsible for complex cognitive processing—shows decreased activity on functional MRI scans during sleep deprivation [10]. These neural changes translate into practical consequences: physicians working more than 24 h make 36% more medical errors than well-rested counterparts [11]. Sleep-deprived physicians take longer to interpret tests and make more errors in diagnostic tasks like X-ray reading [12]. Similar performance declines appear across high-stakes professions—air traffic controllers, emergency responders, and military personnel all show increased error rates with sleep loss.

Historical events demonstrate these effects dramatically. Both the Chernobyl nuclear incident and Space Shuttle Challenger accident involved decisions made by severely sleep-deprived individuals [13]. Current research shows that 24 h of wakefulness produces cognitive impairment equivalent to a blood alcohol concentration of 0.05–0.1%, exceeding legal driving limits in some countries [14]. Even moderate sleep restriction, such as sleeping 6 h per night over 2 weeks, accumulates cognitive deficits, though individuals often fail to recognize these effects [15].

Sleep particularly affects academic performance across all educational levels. Research demonstrates that students who consistently get adequate sleep maintain higher grade point averages, show better information retention, and demonstrate superior problem-solving abilities compared to sleep-deprived peers [16, 17].

Adolescents face unique sleep-related challenges due to their developing brains. During teenage years, the brain undergoes significant rewiring, especially in areas controlling judgment, impulse control, and complex thinking [18]. Sleep-deprived adolescents show decreased activity in the prefrontal cortex, which manages executive functions, and increased activity in reward-seeking brain regions [19]. This imbalance leads to poorer decision-making and increased risk-taking behavior. Their bodies also produce melatonin (the sleep hormone) later in the evening compared to younger children—during puberty, the natural sleep cycle shifts by about 2–3 h later, making it difficult for teenagers to fall asleep before 11 PM or wake refreshed before 8 AM [20].

These biological changes have significant implications for academic scheduling. Schools that start no earlier than 8:30 a.m. see substantial improvements in student outcomes [21]. Studies of school districts with delayed start times report a 4.5% improvement in standardized test scores, 16.5% reduction in traffic accidents involving teen drivers, and a decrease in disciplinary problems [22–24]. Schools that have adjusted their schedules to match adolescent biology also report decreased rates of depression, anxiety, and substance use among students [25]. This biological shift, combined with factors like artificial light exposure and social pressures, makes teenagers particularly vulnerable to chronic sleep deprivation when school schedules don't accommodate their natural sleep patterns.

People often try to compensate for poor sleep (or lack of sleep) through various substances [26]. Alcohol, nicotine, and caffeine might temporarily mask fatigue but typically worsen sleep quality, and not to mention overall health, over time. Caffeine, the most widely used stimulant, blocks adenosine receptors in the brain, temporarily preventing drowsiness but not eliminating the underlying need for sleep. Alcohol might help people fall asleep faster, but it disrupts the natural progression of sleep stages, particularly reducing REM sleep and deep sleep. Nicotine acts as both a stimulant and a sedative, creating irregular sleep patterns and increasing the frequency of nighttime awakenings. The combination of these substances can create complex patterns of sleep disruption that become increasingly difficult to resolve.

The relationship between sleep and cognitive performance is bidirectional—poor sleep affects thinking abilities, and mental strain can disrupt sleep. Intense cognitive activity close to bedtime often makes falling asleep more difficult, despite feeling mentally fatigued. This effect proves particularly strong when engaging in stressful or emotionally charged mental tasks—reviewing work problems, studying for exams, or resolving conflicts—all of which can increase alertness and delay sleep onset. People completing demanding mental tasks before bedtime typically longer to fall asleep and experience more fragmented sleep throughout the night [27]. Long-term sleep deprivation can create lasting changes in cognitive function. Studies of shift workers with more than 10 years of experience show persistent deficits in memory and processing speed, even after returning to regular sleep schedules

[28]. Brain imaging reveals structural changes in white matter—the brain's communication network—suggesting that chronic sleep disruption might cause physical alterations in brain architecture [29]. These findings indicate that while some effects of sleep loss can be reversed with proper rest, long-term sleep disruption might lead to more permanent changes in cognitive capacity.

Research on sleep and cognitive performance raises important implications for workplace safety and public health policy. Studies consistently show that night shift workers have higher rates of errors compared to day shift workers. This risk becomes particularly concerning in sectors where errors can have severe consequences, such as healthcare, transportation, and emergency services. In medical settings, for instance, research demonstrates that extended shifts correlate with increased medical errors, suggesting the need for scheduling practices that ensure adequate rest between shifts. The impact of sleep deprivation extends beyond safety concerns—sleep-deprived workers show higher rates of absenteeism and demonstrate measurable decreases in productivity [30]. Organizations experimenting with later start times or flexible scheduling often report improved work quality and higher employee satisfaction. These findings highlight the potential benefits of workplace policies that better accommodate natural sleep patterns, both for safety and productivity across various industries.

References

1. Cowan N. What are the differences between long-term, short-term, and working memory? Prog Brain. Res 2008;169:323–338. PMID: 18394484.
2. Cleveland Clinic. Short-term memory [Internet]. Cleveland: Cleveland Clinic. Cited 2024 Dec 28. https://my.clevelandclinic.org/health/articles/short-term-memory
3. Almaraz-Espinoza A, Grider MH. Physiology, long term memory. 2023. In: StatPearls [Internet]. Treasure Island: StatPearls; 2025 Jan–. PMID: 31747198.
4. Born J, Wilhelm I. System consolidation of memory during sleep. Psychol Res. 2012;76(2):192–203. PMID: 21541757.
5. Rosinvil T, Lafortune M, Sekerovic Z, Bouchard M, Dubé J, Latulipe-Loiselle A, Martin N, Lina JM, Carrier J. Age-related changes in sleep spindles characteristics during daytime recovery following a 25-hour sleep deprivation. Front Hum Neurosci. 2015;9:323. PMID: 26089788.
6. Walker MP, Brakefield T, Seidman J, Morgan A, Hobson JA, Stickgold R. Sleep and the time course of motor skill learning. Learn Mem 2003;10(4):275–284. PMID: 12888546
7. Killgore WD. Effects of sleep deprivation on cognition. Prog Brain Res. 2010;185:105–129. PMID: 21075236.
8. Guttesen AÁV, Gaskell MG, Madden EV, Appleby G, Cross ZR, Cairney SA. Sleep loss disrupts the neural signature of successful learning. Cereb Cortex. 2023 ;33(5):1610–1625. PMID: 35470400.
9. Corsi-Cabrera M, Ramos J, Arce C, Guevara MA, Ponce-de León M, Lorenzo I. Changes in the waking EEG as a consequence of sleep and sleep deprivation. Sleep. 1992 ;15(6):550–555. PMID: 1475570.
10. Ma N, Dinges DF, Basner M, Rao H. How acute total sleep loss affects the attending brain: a meta-analysis of neuroimaging studies. Sleep. 2015;38(2):233–240. PMID: 25409102.
11. Volpp KG. A delicate balance: physician work hours, patient safety, and organizational efficiency. Circulation. 2008;117(20):2580–2582. PMID: 18490535.
12. Hanna TN, Zygmont ME, Peterson R, Theriot D, Shekhani H, Johnson JO, Krupinski EA. The effects of fatigue from overnight shifts on radiology search patterns and diagnostic performance. J Am Coll Radiol. 2018;15(12):1709–1716. PMID: 29366599.

13. Mitler MM, Carskadon MA, Czeisler CA, Dement WC, Dinges DF, Graeber RC. Catastrophes, sleep, and public policy: consensus report. Sleep. 1988;11(1):100–109. PMID: 3283909.
14. Falleti MG, Maruff P, Collie A, Darby DG, McStephen M. Qualitative similarities in cognitive impairment associated with 24 h of sustained wakefulness and a blood alcohol concentration of 0.05%. J Sleep Res. 2003;12(4):265–274. PMID: 14633237.
15. Yang L, Xi B, Zhao M, Magnussen CG. Association of sleep duration with all-cause and disease-specific mortality in US adults. J Epidemiol Community Health. 2021;jech-2020-215314. PMID: 33441393.
16. Creswell JD, Tumminia MJ, Price S, Sefidgar Y, Cohen S, Ren Y, Brown J, Dey AK, Dutcher JM, Villalba D, Mankoff J, Xu X, Creswell K, Doryab A, Mattingly S, Striegel A, Hachen D, Martinez G, Lovett MC. Nightly sleep duration predicts grade point average in the first year of college. Proc Natl Acad Sci USA 2023;120(8):e2209123120. PMID: 36780521.
17. Princeton University. About the future of families and child wellbeing study [Internet]. Princeton: Princeton University. Cited 2024 Dec 28. https://ffcws.princeton.edu/about
18. Casey BJ, Jones RM, Hare TA. The adolescent brain. Ann N Y Acad Sci. 2008;1124:111–126. PMID: 18400927.
19. Anastasiades PG, de Vivo L, Bellesi M, Jones MW. Adolescent sleep and the foundations of prefrontal cortical development and dysfunction. Prog Neurobiol. 2022;218:102338. PMID: 35963360.
20. American Chemical Society. The science of sleep [Internet]. Washington: ACS. Cited 2024 Dec 28. https://www.acs.org/education/chemmatters/past-issues/archive-2014-2015/the-science-of-sleep.html?t
21. de Araújo LBG, Bianchin S, Pedrazzoli M, Louzada FM, Beijamini F. Multiple positive outcomes of a later school starting time for adolescents. Sleep Health. 2022;8(5):451–457. PMID: 35840536.
22. Dunster GP, de la Iglesia L, Ben-Hamo M, Nave C, Fleischer JG, Panda S, de la Iglesia HO. Sleepmore in Seattle: later school start times are associated with more sleep and better performance in high school students. Sci Adv. 2018;4(12):eaau6200. PMID: 30547089.
23. Danner F, Phillips B. Adolescent sleep, school start times, and teen motor vehicle crashes. J Clin Sleep Med. 2008;4(6):533–535. PMID: 19110880.
24. Thacher PV, Onyper SV. Longitudinal outcomes of start time delay on sleep, behavior, and achievement in high school. Sleep. 2016;39(2):271–281. PMID: 26446106.
25. Berger AT, Widome R, Troxel WM. School start time and psychological health in adolescents. Curr Sleep Med Rep. 2018;4(2):110–117. PMID: 30349805.
26. Spadola CE, Guo N, Johnson DA, Sofer T, Bertisch SM, Jackson CL, Rueschman M, Mittleman MA, Wilson JG, Redline S. Evening intake of alcohol, caffeine, and nicotine: night-to-night associations with sleep duration and continuity among African Americans in the Jackson Heart Sleep Study. Sleep. 2019;42(11):zsz136. PMID: 31386152.
27. Jansen EC, Peterson KE, O'Brien L, Hershner S, Boolani A. Associations between mental workload and sleep quality in a sample of young adults recruited from a US College Town. Behav Sleep Med. 2020;18(4):513–522. PMID: 31220940.
28. Marquié JC, Tucker P, Folkard S, Gentil C, Ansiau D. Chronic effects of shift work on cognition: findings from the VISAT longitudinal study. Occup Environ Med. 2015;72(4):258–264. PMID: 25367246.
29. Grumbach P, Opel N, Martin S, Meinert S, Leehr EJ, Redlich R, Enneking V, Goltermann J, Baune BT, Dannlowski U, Repple J. Sleep duration is associated with white matter microstructure and cognitive performance in healthy adults. Hum Brain Mapp. 2020;41(15):4397–4405. PMID: 32648625.
30. Hafner M, Stepanek M, Taylor J, Troxel WM, van Stolk C. Why sleep matters-the economic costs of insufficient sleep: a cross-country comparative analysis. Rand Health Q. 2017;6(4):11. PMID: 28983434.

Sleep's Role in Mental Health 9

9.1 Sleep and Mental Health: A Two-Way Street

Sleep problems can act as both early warning signs and ongoing symptoms of mental health conditions, while mental health challenges often disrupt sleep patterns [1]. This creates a reinforcing cycle that complicates both diagnosis and treatment.

Sleep disturbances manifest differently across various mental health conditions [1]. In depression, people often experience either excessive sleeping (hypersomnia) or difficulty sleeping (insomnia), frequently waking early and unable to return to sleep [2]. Anxiety commonly disrupts sleep onset—individuals often lie awake with racing thoughts, unable to calm mental activity enough to fall asleep [3]. Bipolar disorder shows distinct sleep patterns: during manic phases, people may feel little need for sleep, while depressive phases often bring profound sleep disruption [4]. In schizophrenia, sleep patterns can become severely disorganized, with disrupted circadian rhythms and fragmented sleep throughout the day and night [5].

The effects of chronic sleep disruption on mental health extend far beyond simple fatigue. When people consistently fail to get adequate sleep, their emotional processing becomes impaired. The amygdala, a brain region crucial for emotional regulation, becomes hyperactive, while the prefrontal cortex, responsible for rational thinking and emotional control, shows reduced function. This biological change may explain why sleep-deprived people often feel more irritable, anxious, and emotionally volatile.

Research reveals that even moderate sleep disruption can significantly affect mental well-being. Even a single night of poor sleep can elevate anxiety levels as much as 30%, while chronic sleep problems raise the risk of developing depression by more than tenfold [6, 7]. These effects stem from sleep's crucial role in emotional processing and stress regulation. During normal sleep, particularly during REM sleep, the brain processes emotional experiences and reduces the intensity of negative memories. Without adequate sleep, emotional memories retain their potency, potentially contributing to anxiety and trauma-related conditions.

A. Juginović, *Sleep Science Made Simple*,
https://doi.org/10.1007/978-3-031-92060-8_9

At the neurobiological level, sleep disruption creates widespread changes in brain chemistry. Poor sleep affects the production and regulation of key neurotransmitters, including serotonin and dopamine, which play crucial roles in mood regulation [7]. The stress hormone cortisol also becomes dysregulated, typically showing elevated levels throughout the day [8]. These neurochemical changes can trigger or worsen mental health symptoms, creating a challenging cycle where poor sleep and mental health problems reinforce each other.

The timing of sleep problems may provide crucial diagnostic clues. Sleep disturbances frequently appear weeks or months before other symptoms of mental health conditions become apparent. For instance, subtle changes in sleep patterns often precede major depressive episodes, while disrupted sleep commonly occurs before manic episodes in bipolar disorder. These early sleep changes may help clinicians identify and possibly prevent the escalation of psychiatric episodes [9].

Improving sleep quality can significantly enhance mental health treatment outcomes. Cognitive-behavioral therapy for insomnia (CBT-I) has shown impressive effectiveness not only for sleep problems but also for concurrent mental health conditions [10]. This specialized therapy helps people identify and change thoughts and behaviors that interfere with sleep, often leading to improvements in both sleep and mental health symptoms. Studies using polysomnography—a comprehensive sleep monitoring technique—show that successful CBT-I treatment increases both total sleep time and sleep efficiency while reducing nocturnal awakening. For people with depression, maintaining regular sleep patterns proves particularly crucial—stable sleep often helps reduce the risk of mood episodes and reduces their severity when they do occur.

The relationship between sleep and mental health extends to medication treatment as well. Many psychiatric medications affect sleep patterns, either improving or disrupting them [11]. Understanding these effects helps clinicians make more informed medication choices. Some antidepressants, for example, can initially disrupt sleep but ultimately lead to more stable sleep patterns as depression improves. Selective serotonin reuptake inhibitors (SSRIs), a commonly used group of antidepressants, often suppress REM sleep initially—a change visible on sleep studies—but this suppression typically normalizes over several weeks as the medication's therapeutic effects emerge. Other medications might help with sleep initially but require careful monitoring to prevent dependency or tolerance. Benzodiazepines, i.e., frequently prescribed sleep medications, can alter natural sleep architecture, reducing time spent in deep sleep stages and potentially compromising sleep's restorative functions [12]. This does not imply that such medications should be avoided, but rather that clinicians and patients should remain aware of the impact these drugs can have on sleep.

Recent research has also revealed the importance of circadian rhythm regulation in mental health treatment [13]. Many mental health conditions involve disrupted circadian rhythms, affecting not just sleep but also appetite, energy levels, and mood throughout the day. Treatments that help stabilize these daily rhythms, such as light therapy or social rhythm therapy, often improve both sleep and mental health symptoms. The implications of this research extend to preventive mental health care.

Protecting sleep quality may help prevent the onset or reduce the severity of mental health conditions in vulnerable individuals. This led to increased emphasis on sleep hygiene in mental health treatment programs and a growing recognition that addressing sleep problems early may help prevent more serious mental health challenges from developing.

9.1.1 Sleep and Depression

Depression ranks among the most prevalent mental health challenges worldwide, affecting approximately 5% of adults according to World Health Organization statistics [14]. Up to 90% of individuals with depression experience significant sleep problems, ranging from difficulty falling asleep to disrupted sleep patterns and early morning awakening [15]. These sleep disturbances create a troubling cycle where poor sleep worsens depressive symptoms, while depression itself further impairs the ability to achieve restorative sleep.

Sleep disruption often appears before other depressive symptoms become apparent [9]. Research shows that individuals with chronic sleep problems, particularly insomnia, face a significantly higher risk of developing depression compared to those who sleep well. This finding positions sleep disturbance not just as a symptom but as a potential early warning sign and risk factor for depression. These early sleep changes manifest in several distinct patterns. Some people experience difficulty falling asleep despite physical tiredness, while others wake frequently throughout the night or early morning. Sleep quality may also decline—individuals often report unrefreshing sleep and persistent fatigue, even when total sleep duration appears adequate. The progression typically begins with intermittent sleep problems that gradually become more persistent. Many individuals first notice changes in their sleep timing, finding themselves either staying awake later or waking earlier than usual. As these disruptions continue, other symptoms begin to emerge—subtle changes in appetite, reduced interest in activities, and mild mood fluctuations, often initially attributed to poor sleep rather than emerging depression.

The intersection of sleep and depression treatment adds further complexity [11]. While antidepressant medications effectively address many depressive symptoms, their impact on sleep varies significantly. SSRIs (selective serotonin reuptake inhibitors), the most commonly prescribed antidepressants, can initially disrupt sleep patterns, particularly during the first couple of weeks of treatment. These medications affect neurotransmitter systems that regulate both mood and sleep-wake cycles, particularly serotonin pathways in the raphe nuclei—a cluster of neurons in the brain stem crucial for sleep regulation. While mood improvements typically take 4–6 weeks to emerge as serotonin receptors gradually adapt, sleep disruption often occurs within days of starting treatment. Some patients report increased difficulty falling asleep or maintaining sleep throughout the night, reflecting these medications' effects on sleep architecture and REM sleep patterns. Other medications, including tricyclic antidepressants and certain SNRIs (serotonin-norepinephrine reuptake inhibitors), often have sedating effects due to their additional impact on histamine and norepinephrine systems in the brain. While this sedation might help some patients sleep, it can lead to persistent daytime drowsiness and alter natural sleep patterns, particularly affecting the duration and timing of different sleep stages.

Treatment approaches increasingly recognize sleep as a crucial component of depression recovery [10]. Cognitive-behavioral therapy for insomnia (CBT-I) has demonstrated particular effectiveness, often improving both sleep quality and mood symptoms simultaneously. This specialized therapy helps individuals identify and modify thoughts and behaviors that interfere with sleep, while also addressing depression-related factors that impair sleep. When combined with traditional depression treatments like psychotherapy and medication, sleep interventions can significantly enhance overall treatment effectiveness. Certain antidepressants, particularly sedating ones like trazodone, doxpein and mirtazapine, are frequently prescribed specifically for their sleep-promoting effects, even in lower doses than typically used for depression—their effects on both mood and sleep providing dual therapeutic benefits. This treatment approach recognizes that improving sleep often serves as a crucial step in breaking the cycle of depression, with better sleep leading to improved mood regulation and enhanced response to other therapeutic interventions.

9.1.2 Sleep and Anxiety

Anxiety disorders affect approximately 20% of adults annually, making them among the most prevalent mental health conditions [16]. Between 60% and 70% of people with anxiety disorders experience significant sleep problems [17]. Individuals with anxiety often struggle to fall asleep, maintain sleep throughout the night, or experience disturbing dreams that fragment their rest. This creates a self-reinforcing pattern where anxiety disrupts sleep, and insufficient sleep then amplifies anxiety symptoms.

Sleep loss can produce immediate and profound effects on anxiety [3]. Research has shown that even a single night of insufficient sleep can significantly increase anxiety symptoms [18]. During sleep deprivation, the brain's emotional centers become hyperactive while regions responsible for rational thinking and emotional control show reduced activity. These brain changes help explain why sleep-deprived individuals often feel more anxious, irritable, and less capable of managing daily stress.

The biological connection between sleep and anxiety involves specific brain regions and neurotransmitter systems [3]. The amygdala, often called the brain's emotion center, becomes hyperreactive during sleep deprivation. Meanwhile, the prefrontal cortex, which normally helps regulate emotional responses, shows decreased activity. Sleep disruption also affects crucial neurotransmitters, including serotonin and GABA (gamma-aminobutyric acid), that typically help regulate anxiety. These changes can create a state of hyperarousal—a persistent alertness that makes relaxation and sleep particularly challenging for people with anxiety disorders.

Enhancing sleep quality often leads to reduced anxiety symptoms, suggesting that sleep interventions should be integral to anxiety treatment [3]. When people with anxiety disorders enhance their sleep, they typically experience better emotional regulation, improved stress resilience, and reduced anxiety levels. Treatment approaches that combine traditional anxiety interventions with sleep-focused strategies, such as CBT-I or relaxation techniques, often yield better outcomes than treating anxiety alone. Sleep disruption often intensifies before periods of increased anxiety, making it a potential early warning sign for anxiety episodes.

9.1.3 Sleep and Bipolar Disorder

Individuals with bipolar disorder experience a complex relationship with sleep, marked by various disturbances including insomnia, excessive sleeping (hypersomnia), and disrupted daily rhythms [4]. These sleep disturbances do more than accompany mood shifts—they can actively trigger manic or depressive episodes, significantly affecting the course of the illness. Bipolar disorder is closely linked to irregularities in circadian rhythms, our internal biological clock that regulates sleep-wake cycles.

Sleep disruptions often emerge as early warning signs of impending mood episodes [4]. At the onset of mania, individuals often experience a sudden drop in sleep need, sometimes sleeping as little as 2 or 3 h while feeling energetic and alert. Conversely, the approach of a depressive episode might bring either excessive sleeping or severe insomnia. These changes in sleep patterns frequently appear days or even weeks before other mood symptoms become apparent, making sleep monitoring a crucial tool in managing bipolar disorder.

Medications used to treat bipolar disorder further complicate sleep management [4]. Mood stabilizers like lithium can help normalize sleep patterns over time, but their effects vary significantly from person to person. Some people experience sleepiness when first starting these medications—a side effect that usually improves with time—while others might develop ongoing sleep difficulties. Antipsychotic medications, commonly used to manage mania, influence multiple brain systems involved in sleep regulation. These medications reduce brain activity by blocking dopamine—a chemical that promotes wakefulness—while also affecting other brain chemicals like serotonin and histamine that influence sleep. As a result, individuals may sleep longer but experience altered sleep architecture, especially in REM sleep.

9.1.4 Sleep and Schizophrenia

Schizophrenia, characterized by hallucinations, delusions, and disorganized thinking, is associated with unusually high rates of sleep disturbances [5]. These sleep problems extend beyond simple insomnia or excessive sleeping (hypersomnia)—they often involve fundamental changes in sleep architecture, the basic organization of sleep stages throughout the night.

The relationship between sleep and schizophrenia symptoms works in both directions. Poor sleep can worsen hallucinations and paranoid thoughts, while psychotic symptoms often make it difficult to maintain regular sleep patterns. This bidirectional cycle complicates treatment, as poor sleep exacerbates psychotic symptoms and those symptoms, in turn, disrupt sleep.

Antipsychotic medications, the primary treatment for schizophrenia, have a major influence on sleep architecture and quality [5]. First-generation (typical) antipsychotics like haloperidol often increase the time it takes to fall asleep and reduce overall sleep efficiency. Second-generation (atypical) antipsychotics generally show more favorable effects on sleep. Medications like clozapine and olanzapine tend to improve sleep architecture by increasing deep sleep and reducing sleep fragmentation. However, these benefits come with potential drawbacks—many patients experience significant daytime drowsiness, and the metabolic changes these medications can cause might indirectly affect sleep quality.

Recent research suggests that addressing sleep problems in schizophrenia might improve overall treatment outcomes [5]. Sleep interventions are increasingly becoming important adjuncts to standard care. These might include specialized cognitive behavioral therapy for sleep problems, education about sleep hygiene, and careful attention to the timing of daily activities. Some clinics now use light therapy and structured daily schedules to help stabilize sleep-wake patterns.

Sedating medications often work better when taken in the evening, helping to promote sleep while minimizing daytime drowsiness. More activating medications might be better taken in the morning to avoid sleep disruption.

References

1. Palagini L, Hertenstein E, Riemann D, Nissen C. Sleep, insomnia and mental health. J Sleep Res. 2022;31(4):e13628. PMID: 35506356.
2. Riemann D, Krone LB, Wulff K, Nissen C. Sleep, insomnia, and depression. Neuropsychopharmacology. 2020;45(1):74–89. PMID: 31071719.
3. Chellappa SL, Aeschbach D. Sleep and anxiety: from mechanisms to interventions. Sleep Med Rev. 2022;61:101583. PMID: 34979437.
4. Morton E, Murray G. An update on sleep in bipolar disorders: presentation, comorbidities, temporal relationships and treatment. Curr Opin Psychol. 2020;34:1–6. PMID: 31521023.
5. Chan MS, Chung KF, Yung KP, Yeung WF. Sleep in schizophrenia: a systematic review and meta-analysis of polysomnographic findings in case-control studies. Sleep Med Rev. 2017;32:69–84. PMID: 27061476.
6. Johns Hopkins Medicine. Depression and sleep: understanding the connection [Internet]. Baltimore: Johns Hopkins Medicine. Cited 2024 Dec 28. https://www.hopkinsmedicine.org/health/wellness-and-prevention/depression-and-sleep-understanding-the-connection
7. Siegel JM. The neurotransmitters of sleep. J Clin Psychiatry. 2004;65(Suppl 16):4–7. PMID: 15575797. PMCID: PMC8761080.
8. Hirotsu C, Tufik S, Andersen ML. Interactions between sleep, stress, and metabolism: from physiological to pathological conditions. Sleep Sci. 2015;8(3):143–152. PMID: 26779321.

9. Franzen PL, Buysse DJ. Sleep disturbances and depression: risk relationships for subsequent depression and therapeutic implications. Dialogues Clin Neurosci. 2008;10(4):473–481. PMID: 19170404.
10. Hertenstein E, Trinca E, Wunderlin M, Schneider CL, Züst MA, Fehér KD, Su T, Straten AV, Berger T, Baglioni C, Johann A, Spiegelhalder K, Riemann D, Feige B, Nissen C. Cognitive behavioral therapy for insomnia in patients with mental disorders and comorbid insomnia: a systematic review and meta-analysis. Sleep Med Rev. 2022;62:101597. PMID: 35240417.
11. Doghramji K, Jangro WC. Adverse effects of psychotropic medications on sleep. Psychiatr Clin North Am. 2016;39(3):487–502. PMID: 27514301.
12. de Mendonça FMR, de Mendonça GPRR, Souza LC, Galvão LP, Paiva HS, de Azevedo Marques Périco C, Torales J, Ventriglio A, Castaldelli-Maia JM, Sousa Martins Silva A. Benzodiazepines and sleep architecture: a systematic review. CNS Neurol Disord Drug Targets. 2023;22(2):172–179. PMID: 34145997.
13. Walker WH 2nd, Walton JC, DeVries AC, Nelson RJ. Circadian rhythm disruption and mental health. Transl Psychiatry. 2020;10(1):28. PMID: 32066704.
14. World Health Organization. Depressive disorder (depression) [Internet]. Geneva: WHO. Cited 2024 Dec 28. https://knowledge-action-portal.com/en/content/depressive-disorder-depression
15. Stickley A, Leinsalu M, DeVylder JE, Inoue Y, Koyanagi A. Sleep problems and depression among 237 023 community-dwelling adults in 46 low- and middle-income countries. Sci Rep. 2019;9(1):12011. PMID: 31427590.
16. Munir S, Takov V. Generalized anxiety disorder. [Updated 2022 Oct 17]. In: StatPearls [Internet]. Treasure Island: StatPearls; 2025 Jan-. https://www.ncbi.nlm.nih.gov/books/NBK441870/
17. Staner L. Sleep and anxiety disorders. Dialogues Clin Neurosci. 2003;5(3):249–258. PMID: 22033804.
18. UC Berkeley News. Stressed to the max? Deep sleep can rewire the anxious brain [Internet]. Berkeley: University of California Berkeley. Cited 2024 Dec 28. https://news.berkeley.edu/2019/11/04/deep-sleep-can-rewire-the-anxious-brain/

Stress, Sleep, and the Body's Adaptive Response

10

10.1 Sleep and Stress: A Vicious Cycle

Sleep and stress interact through multiple biological pathways that significantly affect health [1]. Stress and sleep influence each other continuously: stress can disrupt sleep, while poor sleep increases the body's stress response. This two-way relationship creates patterns that can affect both physical and mental well-being. Studies show that people experiencing high levels of stress often report changes in their sleep patterns, including difficulty falling asleep, frequent night wakings, and poor sleep quality. These sleep disruptions can begin within hours of a stressful event and may persist for weeks or months if the stress continues.

Stress significantly affects our ability to sleep through direct effects on the body's biological systems, particularly the hypothalamic-pituitary-adrenal (HPA) axis—our central stress response system. The HPA axis is the body's main stress management network that connects your brain to hormone-producing glands. When triggered by stress, it releases cortisol (often called the "stress hormone") and other chemicals that keep us alert and vigilant—producing a state of alertness that interferes with the relaxation needed for sleep (Fig. 10.1) [1]. During stress our heart rate rises, muscles become tense, and the mind remains active. This heightened state can persist for hours after a stressful event, making it difficult to relax and fall asleep. Even after the immediate stress passes, the body often maintains this state of heightened alertness, leading to sleep difficulties. When stress becomes an ongoing issue, these disruptions can create persistent sleep problems, including trouble falling asleep, frequent nighttime awakenings, and poor sleep quality. The relationship works both ways—poor sleep increases sensitivity to stress, creating a cycle that can become increasingly difficult to break without addressing both the stress and sleep components.

Brain imaging studies reveal how stress affects sleep-related brain activity [1, 2]. Stress increases activity in brain regions involved in emotional processing and alertness while decreasing activity in areas that promote sleep and relaxation. Using functional magnetic resonance imaging (fMRI) that infers neuronal activity by

A. Juginović, *Sleep Science Made Simple*,
https://doi.org/10.1007/978-3-031-92060-8_10

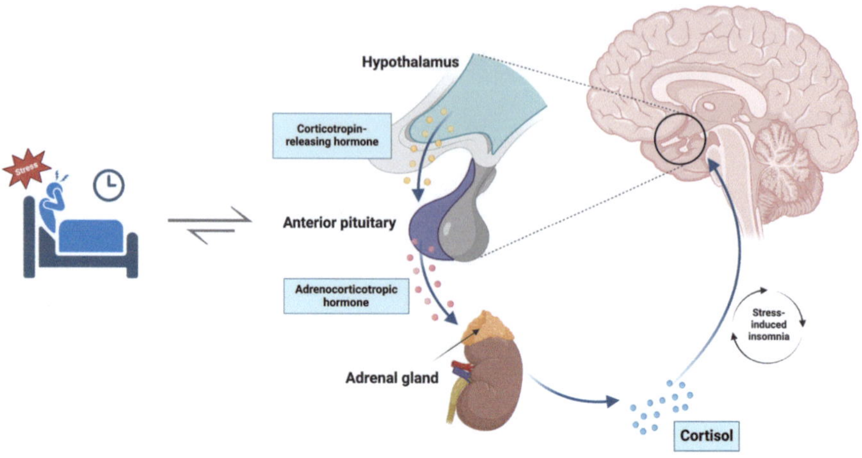

Fig. 10.1 The hypothalamic-pituitary-adrenal (HPA) axis: stress response mechanism. ("Created in BioRender. Juginovic, A. (2025) https://BioRender.com/t71h717")

measuring changes in blood flow, researchers have observed that stressed individuals show heightened activity in the amygdala, the brain's "alarm center" responsible for detecting threat and emotional salience. At the same time, activity in the prefrontal cortex, which helps regulate emotional responses, becomes reduced. These brain activity changes often outlast the initial stressor, creating a state of hyperarousal that interferes with the natural transition to sleep. Even when people report feeling relatively calm, their brains may continue showing patterns of stress-related activation that make sleep difficult.

The timing of stress exposure particularly affects sleep quality [3]. Stress experienced late in the day tends to have stronger effects on sleep than similar stress earlier in the day. This timing effect relates to the body's natural daily rhythms—evening hours normally involve decreasing stress hormone levels to prepare for sleep. Studies show that exposure to stress in the late afternoon or evening can delay the evening decline in cortisol levels which may increase the risk of sleep problems [4]. This disruption affects not only sleep initiation but also the distribution of sleep stages throughout the night. Evening stress increases time spent in lighter sleep stages and reduces deep sleep, resulting in less restorative rest. The effects become even more pronounced when evening stress combines with exposure to artificial light, which can further disrupt the body's natural preparation for sleep.

Work-related stress presents particular challenges for sleep health [5]. Studies of different occupations show that high job stress correlates with increased sleep problems, especially among people who work irregular hours or face high-pressure deadlines. Healthcare workers, emergency responders, and professionals in financial sectors often report significant sleep disruption related to work stress [6]. The combination of long hours, high responsibility, and irregular schedules can create persistent patterns of sleep disruption that affect both job performance and overall health. Organizations that have implemented stress management programs and policies to protect employee sleep often report improvements in both worker well-being and productivity [7].

Long-term activation of stress responses can create persistent changes in sleep patterns [8]. People under chronic stress often develop sleep disorders such as insomnia or sleep-disordered breathing. These conditions can then create additional stress, establishing a cycle where poor sleep and stress continually worsen each other. Research shows that individuals experiencing chronic stress have altered sleep architecture, spending less time in deep sleep and REM sleep—the stages most important for physical and mental restoration [9]. This reduction in restorative sleep can affect everything from immune function to emotional regulation, potentially leading to health consequences that persist even after stress is alleviated.

The connection between sleep and stress extends into the immune system and psychological health [10]. Chronic sleep problems can weaken immune function, making people more susceptible to illness. Studies show that sleep-deprived individuals produce fewer natural killer cells, which help fight off infections and cancer cells [11]. Poor sleep also affects emotional regulation, often leading to increased anxiety and higher risk of depression. The areas of the brain responsible for emotional control, particularly the amygdala and prefrontal cortex, show altered activity patterns after sleep loss. These changes can make people more reactive to negative experiences and less able to regulate their emotional responses, creating a state of psychological vulnerability that can increase sensitivity to stress.

Treatment approaches for sleep and stress problems often work best when addressing both issues together [12]. Cognitive-behavioral therapy for insomnia (CBT-I) helps people identify and change thoughts and behaviors that interfere with sleep while also teaching stress management techniques. This approach typically includes several components: sleep restriction therapy to consolidate sleep into a shorter, more efficient period; stimulus control to strengthen the association between bed and sleep; and cognitive restructuring to address anxiety-producing thoughts about sleep. Studies show that CBT-I can reduce the time it takes to fall asleep by an average of 30–45 minutes and increase total sleep time by 30 min per night [12].

Mindfulness-based stress reduction programs have also proven effective in improving sleep and managing stress [13]. These programs teach techniques that help quiet mental pre-sleep arousal, change unhelpful thoughts about sleep, and build resilience to stress. Regular practice of these techniques can help break the cycle of stress and poor sleep. Studies of mindfulness programs show that participants experience an average reduction of about 20 min in the time it takes to fall asleep, along with improvements in sleep quality and daytime functioning [14]. The benefits extend beyond sleep, with participants reporting reduced anxiety levels, lower blood pressure readings, and better ability to handle stressful situations. These improvements often persist months after completing the program, suggesting that mindfulness training creates lasting changes in how people respond to stress.

References

1. Nollet M, Wisden W, Franks NP. Sleep deprivation and stress: a reciprocal relationship. Interface Focus. 2020;10(3):20190092.
2. Berretz G, Packheiser J, Kumsta R, Wolf OT, Ocklenburg S. The brain under stress-a systematic review and activation likelihood estimation meta-analysis of changes in BOLD signal associated with acute stress exposure. Neurosci Biobehav Rev. 2021;124:89–99. PMID: 33497786.
3. Kalmbach DA, Anderson JR, Drake CL. The impact of stress on sleep: pathogenic sleep reactivity as a vulnerability to insomnia and circadian disorders. J Sleep Res. 2018;27(6):e12710. PMID: 29797753.
4. O'Byrne NA, Yuen F, Butt WZ, Liu PY. Sleep and circadian regulation of cortisol: a short review. Curr Opin Endocr Metab Res. 2021;18:178–186. PMID: 35128146.
5. Mao Y, Raju G, Zabidi MA. Association between occupational stress and sleep quality: a systematic review. Nat Sci Sleep. 2023;15:931–947. PMID: 38021213.
6. Saintila J, Soriano-Moreno AN, Ramos-Vera C, Oblitas-Guerrero SM, Calizaya-Milla YE. Association between sleep duration and burnout in healthcare professionals: a cross-sectional survey. Front Public Health. 2024;11:1268164. PMID: 38269387.
7. Robbins R, Jackson CL, Underwood P, Vieira D, Jean-Louis G, Buxton OM. Employee sleep and workplace health promotion: a systematic review. Am J Health Promot. 2019;33(7):1009–1019 PMID: 30957509.
8. Vgontzas AN, Tsigos C, Bixler EO, Stratakis CA, Zachman K, Kales A, Vela-Bueno A, Chrousos GP. Chronic insomnia and activity of the stress system: a preliminary study. J Psychosom Res. 1998;45(1):21–31. PMID: 9720852.
9. Kim EJ, Dimsdale JE. The effect of psychosocial stress on sleep: a review of polysomnographic evidence. Behav Sleep Med. 2007;5(4):256–278. PMID: 17937582.
10. Segerstrom SC, Miller GE. Psychological stress and the human immune system: a meta-analytic study of 30 years of inquiry. Psychol Bull. 2004;130(4):601–630. PMID: 15250815.
11. De Lorenzo BH, de Oliveira Marchioro L, Greco CR, Suchecki D. Sleep-deprivation reduces NK cell number and function mediated by β-adrenergic signalling. Psychoneuroendocrinology. 2015;57:134–143. PMID: 25929826.
12. Muench A, Vargas I, Grandner MA, Ellis JG, Posner D, Bastien CH, Drummond SP, Perlis ML. We know CBT-I works, now what? Fac Rev. 2022;11:4. PMCID: PMC8808745.
13. Marciniak R, Šumec R, Vyhnálek M, Bendíčková K, Lázničková P, Forte G, Jeleník A, Římalová V, Frič J, Hort J, Sheardová K. The effect of mindfulness-based stress reduction (MBSR) on depression, cognition, and immunity in mild cognitive impairment: a pilot feasibility study. Clin Interv Aging. PMID: 32848377.
14. González-Martín AM, Aibar-Almazán A, Rivas-Campo Y, Marín-Gutiérrez A, Castellote-Caballero Y. Effects of mindfulness-based cognitive therapy on older adults with sleep disorders: a systematic review and meta-analysis. Front Public Health. 2023;11:1242868. PMID: 38179560.

Immunity and Rest

11

11.1 Sleep and Immune Function: A Critical Partnership

Sleep involves more than rest—it actively boosts our immune system [1]. During sleep, the immune system carries out essential maintenance and defense processes that help protect our health. The relationship between sleep and immunity becomes clear when we examine their daily patterns: both follow 24-h cycles, with certain immune cells increasing during night hours while others become more active during the day. This timing isn't coincidental—complex signaling pathways connect our sleep-wake cycles with immune system regulation, though the exact mechanisms continue to be studied.

During sleep, multiple immune processes activate according to specific biological timing. Deep sleep triggers the release of signaling molecules called cytokines that coordinate immune responses [1]. These proteins operate in precise patterns throughout the night, with interleukin-1, interleukin-6, and tumor necrosis factor-alpha showing distinct release cycles. The same period sees increased production of antibodies—proteins that identify and neutralize threats—while regulating white blood cells, particularly natural killer cells and T lymphocytes that defend against pathogens.

Even minor sleep disruptions can alter immune cell production and function significantly, whereas sleep deprivation substantially compromises these immune processes. Studies show that sleeping less than 7 h per night triples susceptibility to the common cold virus compared to longer sleep durations [2]. The risks increase with further sleep loss—individuals getting less than 5 h face a 70% higher risk of pneumonia compared to those achieving 8 h or more [3]. These increased risks stem from measurable decreases in cytokine and antibody production, weakening the immune system's ability to mount effective responses. These immune deficits can persist for days after sleep returns to normal, suggesting longer-term effects.

Sleep affects vaccine responses and immunological memory in several distinct ways [4]. People who get adequate sleep in the days following vaccination develop

A. Juginović, *Sleep Science Made Simple*,
https://doi.org/10.1007/978-3-031-92060-8_11

twice the number of protective antibodies compared to those who don't sleep well. This enhancement stems from sleep's effects on multiple immune components: T helper cells show increased activation, B cells produce antibodies more efficiently, and specific immune proteins that support long-term immunity reach higher levels. These processes don't just improve vaccine responses—they maintain immunity against previously encountered pathogens, explaining why poor sleep often correlates with increased susceptibility to recurring infections.

Sleep quality influences inflammation patterns throughout the body, with particularly notable effects in the digestive system. Poor sleep raises pro-inflammatory molecules in the blood [5]. These elevated inflammatory markers—including C-reactive protein and interleukin-6—often persist throughout the day, creating a state of chronic low-grade inflammation. Studies show that disrupted sleep architecture, particularly reduced slow-wave sleep, correlates with these inflammatory changes [6]. This connection explains why people with consistent sleep problems show higher rates of inflammatory conditions. Studies tracking patients with Crohn's disease (a chronic inflammatory condition affecting any part of the digestive tract), ulcerative colitis (inflammation specifically in the large intestine and rectum) and gastroesophageal reflux disease (GERD; where stomach acid frequently flows back into the esophagus) demonstrate that sleep disruption often precedes symptom flares [7]. The relationship works both ways—inflammatory conditions can disrupt sleep patterns, creating a cycle that proves particularly challenging to break without addressing both components simultaneously.

The gut microbiome—the vast community of bacteria residing in our digestive system—shows surprising sensitivity to sleep patterns [8]. Sleep disruption alters the composition of these bacterial populations in measurable ways, leading to changes in immune system function. This imbalance in gut bacteria may affect both immune function and how we sleep.

The effects of sleep-related inflammation extend far beyond the digestive system. Poor sleep triggers a state of chronic low-grade inflammation throughout the body, measured through elevated inflammatory markers in the blood. These persistent inflammatory changes contribute to the development of cardiovascular disease, alter metabolic processes, and accelerate cellular aging—topics we'll examine in detail in subsequent chapters.

References

1. Besedovsky L, Lange T, Born J. Sleep and immune function. Pflugers Arch. 2012;463(1):121–137. https://doi.org/10.1007/s00424-011-1044-0. PMID: 22071480.
2. Cohen S, Doyle WJ, Alper CM, Janicki-Deverts D, Turner RB. Sleep habits and susceptibility to the common cold. Arch Intern Med. 2009;169(1):62–67. PMID: 19139325.
3. Patel SR, Malhotra A, Gao X, Hu FB, Neuman MI, Fawzi WW. A prospective study of sleep duration and pneumonia risk in women. Sleep. 2012;35(1):97–101. PMID: 22215923.
4. Rayatdoost E, Rahmanian M, Sanie MS, Rahmanian J, Matin S, Kalani N, Kenarkoohi A, Falahi S, Abdoli A. Sufficient sleep, time of vaccination, and vaccine efficacy: a systematic review of the current evidence and a proposal for COVID-19 vaccination. Yale J Biol Med. 2022;95(2):221–235. PMID: 35782481.

5. McEwen BS, Karatsoreos IN. Sleep deprivation and circadian disruption: stress, allostasis, and allostatic load. Sleep Med Clin. 2015;10(1):1–10. PMID: 26055668.
6. Strumberger MA, Häberling I, Emery S, Albermann M, Baumgartner N, Pedrett C, Wild S, Contin-Waldvogel B, Walitza S, Berger G, Schmeck K, Cajochen C. Inverse association between slow-wave sleep and low-grade inflammation in children and adolescents with major depressive disorder. Sleep Med. 2024;119:103–113. PMID: 38669833.
7. Tang Y, Preuss F, Turek FW, Jakate S, Keshavarzian A. Sleep deprivation worsens inflammation and delays recovery in a mouse model of colitis. Sleep Med. 2009;10(6):597–603. https://doi.org/10.1016/j.sleep.2008.12.009. PMID: 19403332.
8. Sun J, Fang D, Wang Z, Liu Y. Sleep deprivation and gut microbiota dysbiosis: current understandings and implications. Int J Mol Sci. 2023;24(11):9603. PMID: 37298553.

Sleep's Influence on Your Metabolism 12

12.1 Sleep's Impact on Metabolic Health

Sleep plays a central role in how the body processes energy and maintains metabolic balance [1]. When sleep patterns become disrupted, these metabolic processes can be impaired, increasing the risk of conditions like type 2 diabetes and obesity. Even one week of reduced sleep can trigger measurable changes in metabolic function.

Getting less than seven hours of sleep per night raises levels of stress hormones like cortisol, disrupts blood sugar regulation, and reduces the body's sensitivity to insulin—the hormone that helps move glucose into cells for energy [2]. These changes mirror the early stages of diabetes development, highlighting how quickly poor sleep can affect metabolism.

During normal sleep, the body maintains precise control over blood sugar levels. However, when sleep becomes disrupted, cells become less responsive to insulin's effects. This condition, known as insulin resistance, can develop even in healthy people during longer periods of poor sleep [3]. For those who already have diabetes, insufficient sleep can make blood sugar control more difficult, potentially leading to a cycle where poor sleep and diabetes symptoms worsen each other.

Sleep also plays a crucial role in regulating appetite and eating behavior [4]. Two key hormones—leptin and ghrelin—control our feelings of fullness and hunger. Poor sleep decreases leptin, which signals fullness, while increasing ghrelin, which triggers hunger. Research shows that consistently sleeping less than five hours per night can lead to weight gain [5]. This hormonal imbalance helps explain why people often feel hungrier and crave high-calorie foods when sleep deprived. Additionally, short sleep can reduce overall energy expenditure by lowering physical activity levels and altering how the body burns calories.

Our internal biological clock, or circadian rhythm, coordinates these metabolic processes throughout the day and night. This timing system manages not just sleep but also how the body processes sugars, fats, and energy. When people work night shifts or keep irregular schedules, they disrupt this careful timing, increasing their

A. Juginovic, *Sleep Science Made Simple*,
https://doi.org/10.1007/978-3-031-92060-8_12

risk of metabolic problems. This may explain why shift workers show higher rates of diabetes, obesity, and related conditions.

Emerging research also points to the gut microbiome as a key player linking sleep to metabolic health. Sleep deprivation can alter the balance of gut bacteria, favoring species associated with obesity and insulin resistance. These microbial changes may increase inflammation and impair how the body processes fats and sugars, further compounding the metabolic risks of poor sleep.

These findings emphasize why good sleep habits matter for metabolic health. Healthcare providers increasingly recognize that addressing sleep problems should be part of treating conditions like diabetes and obesity. This might involve improving sleep habits, treating sleep disorders, or helping shift workers manage their schedules better. For those who must work irregular hours, like healthcare workers, several strategies can help protect metabolic health. These include carefully timing meals to match the body's natural rhythms, using appropriate lighting to help regulate the biological clock, and creating consistent sleep schedules even on days off. While these strategies can't fully reverse the effects of disrupted sleep, they can help minimize its impact on metabolic health.

References

1. Chasens ER, Imes CC, Kariuki JK, Luyster FS, Morris JL, DiNardo MM, Godzik CM, Jeon B, Yang K. Sleep and metabolic syndrome. Nurs Clin North Am. 2021;56(2):203–17.
2. Sharma S, Kavuru M. Sleep and metabolism: an overview. Int J Endocrinol. 2010;2010:270832. PMID: 20811596.
3. Mesarwi O, Polak J, Jun J, Polotsky VY. Sleep disorders and the development of insulin resistance and obesity. Endocrinol Metab Clin N Am. 2013;42(3):617–634. PMID: 24011890.
4. Greer SM, Goldstein AN, Walker MP. The impact of sleep deprivation on food desire in the human brain. Nat Commun. 2013;4:2259. PMID: 23922121.
5. Patel SR, Hu FB. Short sleep duration and weight gain: a systematic review. Obesity (Silver Spring). 2008;16(3):643–653. PMID: 18239586.

The Role of Sleep in Cardiovascular Health

13

13.1 Sleep and Cardiovascular Health

The cardiovascular system relies on sleep not just for rest, but for critical cardiovascular repair and regulation. Understanding how sleep affects heart health helps explain many common patterns we see in cardiovascular disease, from heart attacks and strokes to chronic high blood pressure.

During healthy sleep, blood pressure naturally drops by 10–20% compared to daytime levels [1]. This nightly dip happens because the parasympathetic nervous system takes over, allowing blood vessels to relax and heart rate to slow. When sleep becomes disrupted, this doesn't happen properly. The sympathetic nervous system—which drives our "fight or flight" response—stays more active than it should. Even after a poor night's sleep, you may feel on edge or notice a faster heartbeat. This reflects your sympathetic nervous system remaining active when it should be winding down.

People who don't experience this normal blood pressure drop during sleep—called "non-dippers" in the medical community—face significantly higher risks of both heart attacks and strokes [1]. This is because their cardiovascular system misses its usual period of rest and recovery. It's like running a machine constantly without ever letting it cool down. Over time, this continuous pressure damages the delicate inner lining of blood vessels, making them more prone to developing atherosclerosis—the buildup of fatty plaques that can trigger heart attacks and strokes.

Sleep also helps regulate a crucial hormone system called RAAS (renin-angiotensin-aldosterone system), a hormone pathway critical for blood pressure control [2]. This system produces a hormone called angiotensin II that makes blood vessels constrict. During proper sleep, RAAS activity decreases. But when sleep suffers, RAAS becomes overactive, leading to tighter blood vessels and higher blood pressure. This explains why people often wake up with elevated blood pressure after a poor night's sleep, and why chronic sleep problems so frequently accompany cardiovascular issues.

A. Juginovic, *Sleep Science Made Simple*,
https://doi.org/10.1007/978-3-031-92060-8_13

Heart attacks and strokes show an intriguing pattern—they occur often in the early morning hours, between 6:00 AM and noon [3]. This timing isn't random. Poor sleep affects not just blood pressure, but also how easily blood forms clots. After insufficient sleep, blood platelets become more "sticky," making clots more likely to form [4]. Combined with the morning surge in blood pressure that naturally occurs upon waking due to increased sympathetic activity, these changes create particularly risky conditions for heart attacks and strokes. The body also experiences a surge in stress hormones during these morning hours, which can further strain an already vulnerable cardiovascular system.

This connection between sleep and cardiovascular health extends beyond just blood pressure and clotting. Sleep also affects how the body handles inflammation and oxidative stress—two processes that play key roles in the development of heart disease. During proper sleep, the body can repair damage from oxidative stress and keep inflammation in check. Without adequate sleep, these protective processes become compromised, accelerating the development of cardiovascular problems.

References

1. Habas E Sr, Akbar RA, Alfitori G, Farfar KL, Habas E, Errayes N, Habas A, Al Adab A, Rayani A, Geryo N, Elzouki AY. Effects of nondipping blood pressure changes: a nephrologist prospect. Cureus. 2023;15(7):e42681. PMID: 37649932.
2. Miller MA, Howarth NE. Sleep and cardiovascular disease. Emerg Top Life Sci. 2023;7(5):457–66. PMID: 38084859.
3. Time Magazine. When are you most likely to have a heart attack? [Internet]. New York: Time USA. Cited 2024 Dec 28. https://time.com/archive/6932713/when-are-you-most-likely-to-have-a-heart-attack/
4. Liu H, Wang G, Luan G, Liu Q. Effects of sleep and sleep deprivation on blood cell count and hemostasis parameters in healthy humans. J Thromb Thrombolysis. 2009;28(1):46–49. PMID: 18597046.

How Sleep Supports Brain Health 14

14.1 Sleep and Brain Health

Sleep problems often appear years before the first symptoms of brain disorders emerge [1]. This isn't coincidental—poor sleep actively contributes to conditions like Alzheimer's and Parkinson's disease, while these diseases in turn make sleep even more difficult to maintain. This two-way relationship helps explain why sleep quality becomes increasingly more important as our brains age.

During sleep, the brain activates its specialized cleaning system, called the glymphatic system, which we covered in earlier chapters [1]. Think of it as the brain's nighttime cleaning crew—the spaces between brain cells actually expand during sleep, allowing cerebrospinal fluid to flow more freely and remove built-up waste products from the brain. This process works effectively during deep sleep, but is also active during wake. (Fig. 14.1). One of its main tasks is clearing away beta-amyloid, a protein that can form problematic clumps in the brain. These clumps form the plaques commonly seen in Alzheimer's disease.

When sleep becomes disrupted, this cleaning system can't function properly. Even a single night of poor sleep leads to increased beta-amyloid levels in the brain [2]. Over time, this creates a troubling cycle—poor sleep leads to more protein buildup, which then makes sleep even more difficult. This cycle may help explain why people with chronic sleep problems face higher risks of developing Alzheimer's disease.

Parkinson's disease shows another intriguing connection of sleep and brain health through a condition called REM sleep behavior disorder (RBD) [3]. During normal REM sleep, our bodies remain still while we dream. But people with RBD physically act out their dreams, sometimes with violent movements. This unusual sleep pattern often appears years before other Parkinson's symptoms emerge—typically 5–10 years earlier. Remarkably, many people who develop RBD eventually show signs of Parkinson's disease or related conditions, making it one of the earliest

A. Juginović, *Sleep Science Made Simple*,
https://doi.org/10.1007/978-3-031-92060-8_14

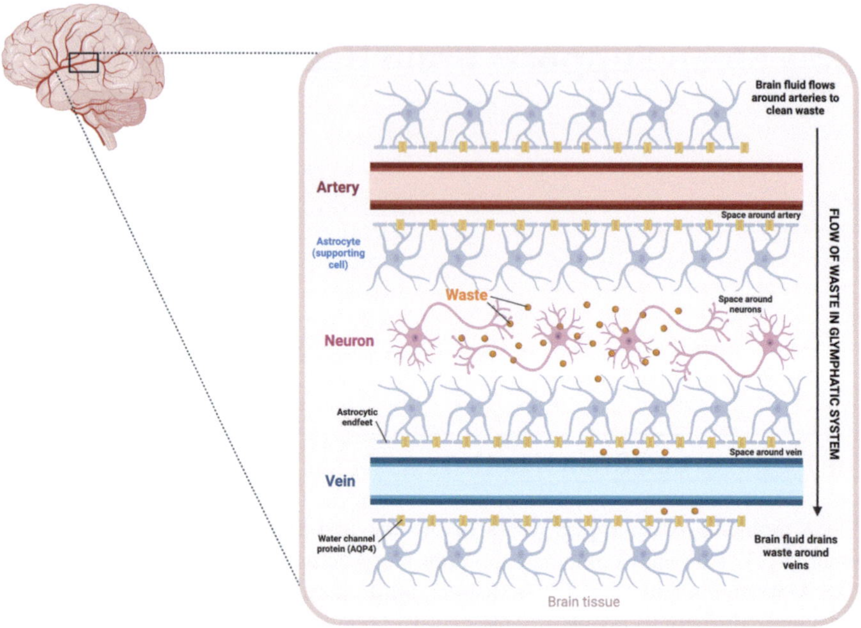

Fig. 14.1 The glymphatic system: brain waste clearance pathway. ("Created in BioRender. Juginovic, A. (2025) https://BioRender.com/r33y434")

warning signs we know of. This early emergence of RBD may reflect changes in brainstem regions also involved in Parkinson's disease.

Poor sleep damages the brain through multiple reinforcing mechanisms [1]. Throughout a sleepless night, inflammation builds up in brain tissue while repair processes slow down. The blood-brain barrier—a protective wall that normally keeps harmful substances out of brain tissue—becomes more permeable, like a fence developing holes. Meanwhile, the production of protective hormones drops, leaving brain cells more vulnerable to damage. Growth hormone, which typically peaks during deep sleep and helps maintain healthy brain tissue, remains at low levels when sleep is disrupted.

Sleep breathing problems create additional risks. In sleep apnea, for instance, the brain experiences hundreds of oxygen drops each night. Each drop forces brain cells into emergency mode—they must work harder with less oxygen, triggering oxidative stress, a process that damages cells through unstable oxygen molecules [4]. Think of trying to run while holding your breath—now imagine your brain cells doing this repeatedly throughout the night. Even mild breathing disruptions can damage sensitive brain regions over time.

These effects become particularly critical during middle age, between 40 and 65 years [5]. During this period, poor sleep habits or untreated sleep disorders can significantly accelerate brain aging. The brain appears especially vulnerable during these years—perhaps because it's already beginning to show subtle age-related changes. Addressing sleep problems during this window becomes crucial for protecting long-term brain health. This is especially evident for conditions like sleep apnea, where each night of untreated breathing problems puts additional strain on an aging brain. We will cover apnea and other sleep disorders in later chapters.

References

1. Bishir M, Bhat A, Essa MM, Ekpo O, Ihunwo AO, Veeraraghavan VP, Mohan SK, Mahalakshmi AM, Ray B, Tuladhar S, Chang S, Chidambaram SB, Sakharkar MK, Guillemin GJ, Qoronfleh MW, Ojcius DM. Sleep deprivation and neurological disorders. Biomed Res Int. 2020;2020:5764017. PMID: 33381558.
2. Shokri-Kojori E, Wang GJ, Wiers CE, Demiral SB, Guo M, Kim SW, Lindgren E, Ramirez V, Zehra A, Freeman C, Miller G, Manza P, Srivastava T, De Santi S, Tomasi D, Benveniste H, Volkow ND. B-Amyloid accumulation in the human brain after one night of sleep deprivation. Proc Natl Acad Sci USA. 2018;115(17):4483–4488. PMID: 29632177.
3. Kim YE, Jeon BS. Clinical implication of REM sleep behavior disorder in Parkinson's disease. J Parkinsons Dis. 2014;4(2):237–244. PMID: 24613864.
4. Yang Q, Wang Y, Feng J, Cao J, Chen B. Intermittent hypoxia from obstructive sleep apnea may cause neuronal impairment and dysfunction in central nervous system: the potential roles played by microglia. Neuropsychiatr Dis Treat. 2013;9:1077–1086. PMID: 23950649.
5. Ramduny J, Bastiani M, Huedepohl R, Sotiropoulos SN, Chechlacz M. The association between inadequate sleep and accelerated brain ageing. Neurobiol Aging. 2022;114:1–14. PMID: 35344818.

15 When Work Disrupts Sleep: Occupational Health Consequences

15.1 Sleep, Shift Work, and Cancer

Sleep's influence on health extends beyond daily functioning and mental clarity. Research reveals significant connections to serious health conditions, including cancer development [1]. Population studies consistently demonstrate links between sleep patterns and cancer risk, with particular evidence for breast and colorectal cancer development [1]. While we observe these connections consistently, it has to be noted that the link is not particularly strong in many studies and the precise biological mechanisms linking sleep to cancer development remain under investigation.

Research reveals specific numbers that help us understand this relationship. In one study, people who regularly slept less than 6 h show a 50% higher rate of colorectal adenomas (early tissue changes that can develop into cancer) [2]. Similarly, women with poor sleep quality face a higher risk of aggressive breast cancer compared to those maintaining healthy sleep patterns [3]. While studies have examined patterns across prostate, lung, and ovarian cancer rates among people with disrupted sleep, the relationship remains complex and not fully understood.

Shift work provides particularly important evidence of how disrupted sleep affects cancer risk [4]. Consider what happens when normal sleep-wake cycles become desynchronized: long-time night shift workers (>15 years) show a 35% higher risk of colorectal cancer and a 9% increase in breast cancer risk compared to people working regular daytime hours [5, 6].

Sleep appears to influence cancer development through several biological mechanisms, though the relationships are complex and still being studied. One factor of interest is melatonin, a hormone that rises at night and helps regulate the body's internal clock. Melatonin may slow tumor growth and reduce oxidative stress [7]. Some studies indicate that people exposed to artificial light at night, such as shift workers, may have lower melatonin levels, which could potentially affect cancer risk [8]. Sleep also appears to support immune system function, which plays a role in identifying and removing abnormal cells. Emerging research suggests that cancer

A. Juginović, *Sleep Science Made Simple*,
https://doi.org/10.1007/978-3-031-92060-8_15

cell activity may vary throughout the day, raising questions about whether the timing of treatments like chemotherapy or radiation could impact their effectiveness. The relationship between sleep and cancer may involve multiple other processes. Poor or insufficient sleep might contribute to chronic inflammation, which could create conditions that affect cancer development [9]. Sleep appears to play a role in DNA repair, which helps prevent mutations, though more research is needed to fully understand this connection [10]. The body's circadian genes, which help regulate cell growth and repair, may also be affected by sleep patterns, though the exact mechanisms aren't fully understood [11]. While poor sleep quality has been associated with increased oxidative stress, which can damage cells and DNA, the direct link to cancer development requires further study [12].

On a surprising note in regard to cancer risk and sleep, a recent study showed that circulating tumor cells (CTCs), which are responsible for cancer's spread throughout the body, are predominantly released during sleep periods [13]. The researchers found that these rest-phase CTCs have a significantly higher capacity to form new tumors compared to those released during waking hours, with genetic analysis revealing increased activity of cell division genes specifically during sleep. This discovery suggests that the most dangerous phase of cancer dissemination may occur during our rest period, adding an unexpected twist to our understanding of sleep's role in cancer progression. These results, while really interesting, still need further validation and research.

References

1. Lingas EC. A narrative review of the carcinogenic effect of night shift and the potential protective role of melatonin. Cureus. 2023;15(8):e43326.
2. Thompson CL, Larkin EK, Patel S, Berger NA, Redline S, Li L. Short duration of sleep increases risk of colorectal adenoma. Cancer. 2011;117(4):841–7. PMID: 20936662.
3. Soucise A, Vaughn C, Thompson CL, Millen AE, Freudenheim JL, Wactawski-Wende J, Phipps AI, Hale L, Qi L, Ochs-Balcom HM. Sleep quality, duration, and breast cancer aggressiveness. Breast Cancer Res Treat. 2017;164(1):169–78. PMID: 28417334.
4. Centers for Disease Control and Prevention (CDC). Recent news about night shift work and cancer: what does it mean for workers? [Internet]. Atlanta: CDC; 2021. Cited 2024 Dec 28. https://blogs.cdc.gov/niosh-science-blog/2021/04/27/nightshift-cancer/
5. Wei F, Chen W, Lin X. Night-shift work, breast cancer incidence, and all-cause mortality: an updated meta-analysis of prospective cohort studies. Sleep Breath. 2022;26(4):1509–26. PMID: 34775538.
6. Schernhammer ES, Laden F, Speizer FE, Willett WC, Hunter DJ, Kawachi I, Fuchs CS, Colditz GA. Night-shift work and risk of colorectal cancer in the nurses' health study. J Natl Cancer Inst. 2003;95(11):825–8. PMID: 12783938.
7. Li Y, Li S, Zhou Y, Meng X, Zhang JJ, Xu DP, Li HB. Melatonin for the prevention and treatment of cancer. Oncotarget. 2017;8(24):39896–921. PMID: 28415828.
8. Mirick DK, Bhatti P, Chen C, Nordt F, Stanczyk FZ, Davis S. Night shift work and levels of 6-sulfatoxymelatonin and cortisol in men. Cancer Epidemiol Biomarkers Prev. 2013;22(6):1079–87. PMID: 23563887.
9. Mullington JM, Simpson NS, Meier-Ewert HK, Haack M. Sleep loss and inflammation. Best Pract Res Clin Endocrinol Metab. 2010 Oct;24(5):775–84. PMID: 21112025.

10. Mourrain P, Wang GX. Sleep: DNA repair function for better neuronal aging? Curr Biol. 2019;29(12):R585–8. PMID: 31211981.
11. Sochal M, Ditmer M, Tarasiuk-Zawadzka A, Binienda A, Turkiewicz S, Wysokiński A, Karuga FF, Białasiewicz P, Fichna J, Gabryelska A. Circadian rhythm genes and their association with sleep and sleep restriction. Int J Mol Sci. 2024;25(19):10445. PMID: 39408776.
12. Gopalakrishnan A, Ji LL, Cirelli C. Sleep deprivation and cellular responses to oxidative stress. Sleep. 2004;27(1):27–35. PMID: 14998234.
13. Diamantopoulou Z, Castro-Giner F, Schwab FD, Foerster C, Saini M, Budinjas S, Strittmatter K, Krol I, Seifert B, Heinzelmann-Schwarz V, Kurzeder C, Rochlitz C, Vetter M, Weber WP, Aceto N. The metastatic spread of breast cancer accelerates during sleep. Nature. 2022;607(7917):156–62. PMID: 35732738.

16 Balancing Between Too Little and Too Much Sleep

16.1 Balancing Sleep: The Risk of Sleep Deprivation and Oversleeping

Many health problems linked to poor sleep raise a fundamental question: can a lack of sleep directly cause death? While human cases of death directly from sleep deprivation remain rare (if any), research provides compelling evidence that prolonged sleep loss in animals can indeed prove fatal.

When rats are prevented from sleeping, they die after about a few weeks [1]. Even more dramatic evidence comes from studies of fruit flies, where just a few days of sleep deprivation triggers a cascade of biological changes that dramatically shorten their lives [2]. The key mechanism appears to involve the buildup of harmful molecules called reactive oxygen species (ROS) not in the brain, but in the small and large intestines. These reactive oxygen species normally serve as important signaling molecules in the body. However, when sleep deprivation prevents their proper clearance, they accumulate to dangerous levels, particularly in the gut. This buildup creates oxidative stress that damages cells' basic components—their proteins, fats, and even DNA [2]. When researchers gave sleep-deprived fruit flies antioxidants to neutralize these harmful molecules, the flies' lifespans returned to normal despite still not sleeping almost at all.

Similar patterns appear in mice, where just 2 days of partial sleep loss leads to increased reactive oxygen species in the digestive system [2]. This damage primarily targets the gut, while other organs show little to no oxidative stress from sleep loss. However, studying long-term survival in mice proves challenging because of their relatively long 2-year lifespan compared to fruit flies, which live only about 40 days.

In humans, our understanding of sleep deprivation's lethal potential comes mainly from studying a rare genetic condition called fatal familial insomnia [3]. This brain disorder causes progressively worsening sleeplessness that leads to death within months to years. The condition primarily affects the thalamus, a brain region

A. Juginovic, *Sleep Science Made Simple*,
https://doi.org/10.1007/978-3-031-92060-8_16

crucial for sleep regulation. However, scientists still debate whether death results directly from sleep loss or from other aspects of the disease.

On the other end of the spectrum, regularly sleeping more than 9–10 h per night may also be associated with negative health outcomes. However, the relationship between extended sleep and health is complex and often bidirectional, making it difficult to determine whether long sleep is a cause or a symptom of poor health.

Observational studies have found associations between long sleep duration and various health conditions, including cardiovascular issues and metabolic changes [4]. However, these relationships may reflect underlying health conditions rather than sleep duration itself causing problems. Most importantly, extended sleep is often a symptom rather than a core problem. Many medical conditions cause people to sleep longer than usual—depression frequently leads to extended sleep as the brain's mood regulation systems become disrupted, while chronic fatigue conditions, autoimmune disorders, thyroid conditions, and certain neurological conditions can all increase sleep duration [4]. Even common conditions like hypothyroidism or iron-deficiency anemia can lead to increased sleep duration through different (and not so clear) mechanisms—low thyroid levels slow down bodily processes while anemia reduces oxygen delivery, both of which may contribute to increased sleep need or fatigue.

Individual sleep needs vary significantly due to genetic factors, age, activity level, and overall health status. Some people naturally require longer sleep durations to feel refreshed, similar to how height varies in the population, but the consensus is that sleeping over 9 h continuously is considered oversleeping. The key distinction is between naturally longer sleep patterns and sudden changes in sleep duration, which may warrant medical attention. Given that extended sleep often signals underlying health changes, it's crucial to investigate unexpected increases in sleep duration with a healthcare provider rather than assuming it's simply a natural variation, especially since many underlying causes like thyroid dysfunction or anemia are readily treatable with appropriate medical care.

References

1. Everson CA, Bergmann BM, Rechtschaffen A. Sleep deprivation in the rat: III. Total sleep deprivation. Sleep. 1989;12(1):13–21. PMID: 2928622.
2. Vaccaro A, Kaplan Dor Y, Nambara K, Pollina EA, Lin C, Greenberg ME, Rogulja D. Sleep loss can cause death through accumulation of reactive oxygen species in the gut. Cell. 2020;181(6):1307–1328.e15. PMID: 32502393.
3. Khan Z, Sankari A, Bollu PC. Fatal familial insomnia. Updated 2024 Feb 25. In: StatPearls [Internet]. Treasure Island: StatPearls; 2025 Jan-. https://www.ncbi.nlm.nih.gov/books/NBK482208/
4. Klerman EB, Barbato G, Czeisler CA, Wehr TA. Can people sleep too much? Effects of extended sleep opportunity on sleep duration and timing. Front Physiol. 2021;12:792942. PMID: 35002775.

17 Sleep's Role in Productivity, Leadership, and Economic Outcomes

17.1 Sleep in the Business World

17.1.1 The High Price of Poor Sleep: Implications for Leadership and the Economy

The demands of modern leadership require quick, complex decisions that shape organizational futures. Research reveals that sleep quality significantly affects how well leaders perform these crucial tasks, influencing everything from strategic thinking to daily decision-making.

The effects of poor sleep on leadership skills are particularly strong. Studies show that sleep-deprived individuals perform at levels similar to those who are legally intoxicated [1]. Their ability to process information, maintain attention, and make sound decisions becomes severely compromised. This finding raises serious concerns in today's business culture, where constant connectivity and rapid growth often create an environment of perpetual urgency. Many managers unknowingly create conditions that harm sleep quality—both for themselves and their teams. Late nights become routine, weekends blur into workdays, and chronic stress becomes the new normal. This environment breeds sleep problems and triggers a cascade of performance issues. When leaders operate under chronic sleep loss, their impaired judgment can gradually guide an organization off course, often without anyone recognizing sleep deprivation as the root cause.

Sleep plays a vital role in how leaders learn and remember information [2]. During sleep, the brain processes information gathered during the day, strengthening important connections and enhancing both memory storage and recall. This process proves especially important for leaders who must maintain and apply complex information when making decisions. Without proper sleep, their ability to absorb new information and retrieve stored knowledge becomes compromised. When leaders operate with insufficient sleep, their impaired judgment and reduced emotional control can affect entire teams. Their decision-making becomes less reliable, their emotional responses more volatile, and their ability to inspire and guide others

A. Juginović, *Sleep Science Made Simple*,
https://doi.org/10.1007/978-3-031-92060-8_17

diminishes. These effects can create a ripple of reduced productivity and effectiveness throughout an organization.

Some leaders attempt to manage sleep deprivation through strategic approaches like taking regular short breaks or delegating tasks. While these strategies can help when sleep loss is unavoidable, they don't replace the fundamental need for adequate sleep. Research consistently shows that leaders who prioritize sleep demonstrate better decision-making capabilities and achieve superior organizational outcomes [2].

The relationship between sleep and leadership effectiveness carries profound implications for organizational success. Leaders must recognize that prioritizing sleep represents more than a personal health choice—it fundamentally affects their ability to guide their organizations effectively. The cognitive impairments associated with sleep loss, comparable to those of intoxication, highlight the critical nature of this issue. Poor sleep affects more than just individual performance—it can shape the entire organization's trajectory.

Beyond the impact on leadership and organizational performance, poor sleep also creates substantial economic costs. In the United States alone, sleep loss costs businesses approximately $400 billion annually through missed workdays, workplace accidents, and reduced productivity [3]. The economic burden of specific sleep disorders is also significant: insomnia costs up to $107 billion yearly, while undiagnosed sleep apnea costs nearly $150 billion annually. Proper diagnosis and treatment of sleep apnea alone could save about $100 billion each year [4, 5].

At the individual level, the financial impact of poor sleep is evident in healthcare costs. People with insomnia spend between $4220 and $5580 more on medical expenses compared to those who sleep well [6]. Employers also face significant costs—each employee with sleep problems costs a company $200–3000 annually in lost productivity alone [6]. For large companies, these losses can be substantial. Even conservative estimates suggest a single large company may lose up to half a million dollars yearly due to sleep-related productivity declines.

The economic effects of poor sleep extend across many industries. In transportation, drowsy driving causes approximately 72,000 car accidents each year, resulting in $12.5 billion in losses, as well as many injuries and even fatalities [7]. Manufacturing companies face costs from fatigue-related machinery accidents, including equipment damage and legal expenses. Service industries see reduced worker productivity and lower service quality, leading to lost revenue and unhappy customers.

However, some companies have found that investing in employee sleep health yields positive returns. Research shows that workplace health programs save $3.27 for every dollar spent, while programs reducing missed workdays save $2.73 per dollar invested [8]. When employees improve their sleep quality, their productivity losses decrease significantly, suggesting that educating workers about good sleep habits can be a worthwhile investment for companies (Fig. 17.1).

Sleep-related economic losses often lurk in unexpected areas. Poor sleep affects decision-making, potentially leading to costly business errors. It reduces creativity and innovation, hindering a company's competitive edge. Customer service quality suffers when tired employees interact with clients. These subtle effects may not be

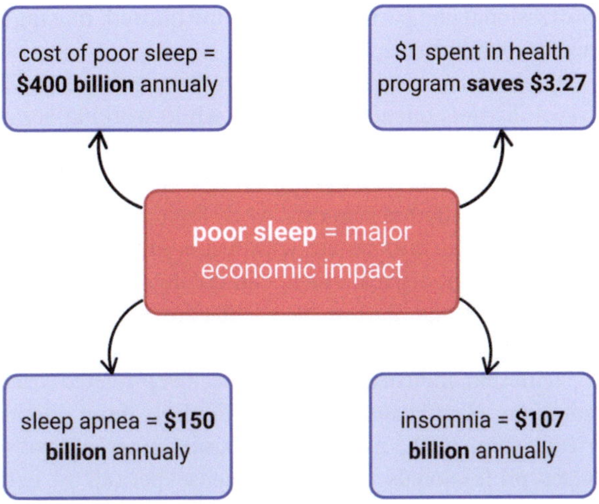

Fig. 17.1 Schematic overview of the hidden cost of poor sleep—how sleep deprivation impacts the economy. ("Image generated by ChatGPT (OpenAI), 2025. Used with permission")

immediately apparent in financial reports, but they significantly impact long-term business success.

In conclusion, sleep deprivation poses a significant threat not only to individual health and leadership effectiveness but also to the economic well-being of businesses and society as a whole. Prioritizing sleep, both at the individual and organizational level, is crucial for optimizing performance, reducing costs, and achieving success in today's demanding world.

17.1.2 From Fatigue to Focus: How Modern Workplaces Can Prioritize Sleep Health

The modern workplace often inadvertently undermines healthy sleep patterns through its underlying culture and unstated expectations. Many organizations unknowingly create environments that discourage proper rest, whether through explicit policies or implicit pressures. When companies expect constant availability or praise employees who work extended hours, they create powerful incentives that work against healthy sleep habits. Some employees report checking work emails until moments before bed and immediately upon waking, disrupting the natural transition periods that help regulate healthy sleep. This "always-on" mentality can significantly impair restorative sleep.

The shift toward remote and hybrid work has presented both opportunities and challenges for sleep health. While eliminating commute times theoretically allows for more sleep, many remote workers find themselves working longer hours and struggling to maintain boundaries between work and rest. The increased reliance on screens for virtual meetings adds another layer of complexity, as extended exposure to blue light from devices can disrupt natural sleep timing. Some people working from home report difficulty "shutting off" at the end of the workday, their minds continuing to process work matters well into evening hours. The lines between professional and personal life become blurred, making it difficult to fully disengage and prepare for sleep.

Global business operations create unique challenges for sleep health. International travel disrupts circadian rhythms, while working across time zones often requires early morning or late evening meetings that conflict with natural sleep patterns. A manager in New York joining a 9 AM meeting in London must wake hours before their natural rhythm suggests, while their colleague in San Francisco might sacrifice evening rest to collaborate with teams in Asia. These disruptions, occurring regularly in global organizations, can create chronic sleep challenges that affect decision-making and performance. The constant shifting of sleep schedules can lead to persistent fatigue and reduced cognitive function.

Different industries face unique sleep-related challenges that require tailored solutions. Healthcare workers, particularly those rotating through night shifts, experience some of the most severe disruptions to natural sleep patterns. Financial services professionals often face intense periods of extended work hours that can destroy sleep routines for weeks at a time. Manufacturing employees working rotating shifts may never fully adapt to changing schedules, their bodies caught in a constant state of circadian misalignment. These industry-specific sleep challenges necessitate targeted interventions and support systems.

Forward-thinking organizations have begun implementing policies that protect and promote healthy sleep. Some companies now restrict after-hours email access, creating technology blackout periods that allow employees to truly disconnect [9]. Others provide education about sleep health and create workplace environments that support proper rest. Dedicated quiet rooms offer spaces for brief restorative naps, while flexible start times accommodate different chronotypes—natural tendencies to be more alert in the morning or evening [10]. Even office lighting has come under scrutiny, with some companies installing systems that change throughout the day to better support natural circadian rhythms. These initiatives demonstrate a growing recognition of sleep's critical role in employee well-being and productivity.

Technology's relationship with workplace sleep proves particularly complex. The same devices that can disrupt sleep through late-night work notifications also offer tools for improving rest. Sleep-tracking applications help people understand their sleep patterns, while screen-filtering software reduces exposure to sleep-disrupting blue light. Organizations may now use specialized lighting systems that adjust throughout the day, supporting natural circadian rhythms even in indoor environments [11]. The key lies in leveraging technology mindfully, minimizing its disruptive potential while maximizing its benefits for sleep health.

The effectiveness of these interventions becomes clear in organizations that prioritize sleep health. Companies implementing comprehensive sleep programs report reduced absenteeism, fewer workplace accidents, and improved employee satisfaction. When organizations acknowledge and address sleep's role in performance, they create environments that support both individual well-being and organizational success. A culture that values sleep fosters a more productive, engaged, and healthy workforce.

Creating meaningful change in organizational sleep health requires more than simply acknowledging the problem. Successful implementation of sleep-friendly practices demands a systematic approach that considers every level of the organization. Companies achieving the greatest success begin by examining their fundamental assumptions about work and productivity, often challenging long-held beliefs about the relationship between hours worked and value created. A shift in mindset is necessary, recognizing that well-rested employees are more efficient and effective than those who are chronically sleep-deprived.

The transition toward better sleep practices often starts with senior leadership publicly acknowledging their own sleep needs and habits. When executives discuss the importance of proper rest and demonstrate through their actions that taking time to sleep represents a priority rather than a weakness, it creates permission throughout the organization for others to do the same. Some companies now include sleep hygiene discussions in their leadership development programs, treating healthy sleep as an essential leadership skill rather than a personal choice. Leaders who prioritize sleep serve as role models, encouraging a culture that values rest and well-being.

The physical workplace itself plays a crucial role in supporting healthy sleep patterns. Organizations can design office spaces that expose employees to natural light throughout the day, helping maintain proper circadian rhythms even during long indoor workdays. Meeting schedules can accommodate different chronotypes and time zones without requiring excessive early morning or late evening commitments. Even small changes, like providing spaces for brief restorative rest periods during the workday, can significantly impact employee well-being and performance. A thoughtfully designed workspace can contribute to a more restful and productive work environment.

Measuring the impact of sleep initiatives proves essential for maintaining organizational commitment. Companies successfully implementing sleep health programs typically track various metrics, from obvious measures like absenteeism and accident rates to subtler indicators such as meeting effectiveness and innovation outputs. Understanding these impacts helps justify continued investment in sleep health while identifying areas needing adjustment or improvement. Data-driven evaluation ensures that sleep health initiatives are effective and aligned with organizational goals.

Sleep health extends beyond individual choice into the realm of organizational responsibility. Just as companies invest in physical safety equipment or mental health resources, they must consider sleep health an essential component of employee well-being and organizational performance. This investment in sleep health, while requiring initial resource commitment, consistently demonstrates positive returns through improved productivity, reduced errors, and enhanced innovation capacity. Prioritizing sleep is not just a perk; it's a strategic investment in a company's most valuable asset: its people.

References

1. Williamson AM, Feyer AM. Moderate sleep deprivation produces impairments in cognitive and motor performance equivalent to legally prescribed levels of alcohol intoxication. Occup Environ Med. 2000;57(10):649–55. PMID: 10984335.

2. Shanafelt T, Trockel M, Rodriguez A, Logan D. Wellness-centered leadership: equipping health care leaders to cultivate physician well-being and professional fulfillment. Acad Med. 2021;96(5):641–51. PMID: 33394666.
3. Hafner M, Stepanek M, Taylor J, Troxel WM, Van Stolk C. Why sleep matters – the economic costs of insufficient sleep: a cross-country comparative analysis [Internet]. Santa Monica: RAND; 2016. Cited 2024 Jan 26. https://www.rand.org/pubs/research_reports/RR1791.html
4. Institute of Medicine (US) Committee on Sleep Medicine and Research, Colten HR, Altevogt BM, editors. Sleep disorders and sleep deprivation: an unmet public health problem. Washington: National Academies Press (US); 2006. 4, Functional and economic impact of sleep loss and sleep-related disorders. https://www.ncbi.nlm.nih.gov/books/NBK19958/
5. American Academy of Sleep Medicine (AASM). Economic burden of undiagnosed sleep apnea in U.S. is nearly $150B per year [Internet]. Darien: AASM; Cited 2024 Jan 26. https://aasm.org/economic-burden-of-undiagnosed-sleep-apnea-in-u-s-is-nearly-150b-per-year/
6. Rosekind MR, Gregory KB, Mallis MM, Brandt SL, Seal B, Lerner D. The cost of poor sleep: workplace productivity loss and associated costs. J Occup Environ Med. 2010;52(1):91–8. PMID: 20042880.
7. National Sleep Foundation (NSF). Sleep first. Drive Alert [Internet]. Washington, DC: NSF; Cited 2024 Dec 26. https://www.thensf.org/drowsy-driving-prevention
8. Chen CY, Schultz AB, Li X, Burton WN. The association between changes in employee sleep and changes in workplace health and economic outcomes. Popul Health Manag. 2018;21(1):46–54. PMID: 28486056.
9. CBS News. The "right to disconnect" from work: More laws are banning after-hours emails and calls [Internet]. New York: CBS Interactive; Cited 2024 Jan 26. https://www.cbsnews.com/news/the-right-to-disconnect-from-work-more-laws-are-banning-after-hours-emails-and-calls/.
10. CommercialCafe. 20 Companies where it's ok to nap [Internet]. CommercialCafe;Cited 2024 Jan 26. https://www.commercialcafe.com/blog/20-companies-where-its-ok-to-nap/
11. Pereira MOK, Almeida BF, Bolzan TE, Pinto RA, Bender VC. Adjustable lighting system based on circadian rhythm for human comfort. J Opt. 2022;51(4):1028–37. PMCID: PMC9112644.

The Crucial Role of Sleep for Athletes 18

18.1 Sleep and Athletes

Sleep profoundly affects athletic performance, from reaction time and accuracy to injury prevention and recovery [1]. Research reveals striking differences between well-rested and sleep-deprived athletes, with sleep quality often making the difference between peak performance and poor results. Modern approaches to measuring individual sleep patterns, including serial melatonin sampling through saliva tests and wearable devices, allow trainers to understand each athlete's unique sleep-wake cycle with unprecedented precision.

Unfortunately, sleep problems affect athletes more often than many realize. Studies show that up to 2/3 of elite athletes report poor sleep quality and 33% struggling with insomnia [1, 2]. These problems often stem from intense training schedules, frequent travel, competition anxiety, and evening electronic device use. Research in pharmacogenomics reveals that some athletes metabolize sleep medications differently based on their genetic makeup, explaining why standard doses might help some athletes while proving ineffective or causing side effects in others.

Even modest sleep loss significantly impacts athletic performance. Losing sleep impairs muscle strength, shooting accuracy, as well as sprint time [1]. Advanced monitoring systems now track subtle changes in performance metrics, allowing early detection of sleep-related decline before it significantly impacts training or competition (Fig. 18.1).

In contrast, proper sleep enhances athletic capabilities. Athletes sleeping eight or more hours nightly show better reaction times, accuracy, and overall physical performance compared to those sleeping less [1]. Adequate sleep also reduces injury risk by a substantial amount [3]. These improvements stem from sleep's essential role in muscle recovery, hormonal regulation, and cognitive functioning. Modern sleep science now enables personalized sleep optimization through detailed analysis of each athlete's sleep architecture, hormonal patterns, and genetic factors affecting sleep medication metabolism.

A. Juginović, *Sleep Science Made Simple*,
https://doi.org/10.1007/978-3-031-92060-8_18

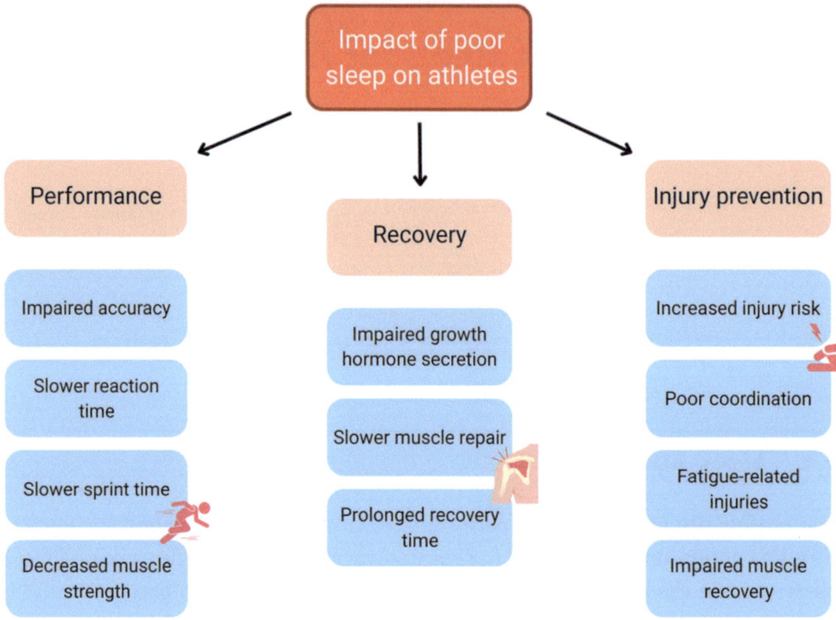

Fig. 18.1 Illustrative overview of how poor sleep undermines athletic performance and injury recovery. ("Image generated by ChatGPT (OpenAI), 2025. Used with permission")

An athlete's natural sleep timing preference, or chronotype, also affects performance [4]. Some athletes naturally perform better in the morning ("larks"), while others peak in the evening ("owls"). Morning-type athletes show superior strength test results early in the day, while evening-types perform better later. Understanding these patterns allows for infividualized training schedules—morning-types might benefit from early training when their alertness peaks, while evening-types might perform better in later sessions. Genetic testing can now identify variations in clock genes that influence these preferences, allowing for more precise training schedule optimization.

The relationship between sleep and injury rehabilitation deserves particular attention. Athletes recovering from injuries show significantly faster healing rates when maintaining optimal sleep patterns [5]. During deep sleep stages, growth hormone secretion peaks, accelerating tissue repair and muscle growth [6]. Inflammatory responses, essential for tissue recovery, also operate more effectively with adequate sleep, potentially speeding up recovery time.

Sleep quality during intensive training periods proves especially important. The brain uses sleep to consolidate new movement patterns and refine athletic skills, making proper rest particularly important when learning new techniques or preparing for competition. Some training centers now adjust training intensity based on sleep quality metrics, reducing workout loads when sleep data indicates insufficient recovery. This strategy helps prevent overtraining syndrome, a state of chronic fatigue and underperformance caused by inadequate recovery between intense training sessions [7].

Travel and competition present particular challenges for athletes' sleep. Crossing time zones disrupts the body's internal clock, reducing alertness and slowing reactions. This jet lag effect can persist for several days, affecting performance and increasing injury risk. Even traveling within the same time zone can disrupt sleep patterns through changes in schedule and environment. New approaches use serial melatonin profiling and personalized light therapy to help athletes adjust their circadian rhythms more quickly when traveling.

The impact of poor sleep extends beyond physical performance. Sleep-deprived athletes often show decreased motivation and resilience while experiencing higher levels of anxiety and depression [1]. These psychological effects can impair focus, motivation, and emotional regulation, proving just as detrimental to performance as physical fatigue, potentially affecting an athlete's entire career.

Athletes can protect their sleep quality through several strategies. Maintaining consistent sleep schedules, even during training periods, helps regulate the body's internal clock. Creating proper sleep environments—dark, quiet, and cool rooms—promotes better rest. When traveling, gradually shifting sleep and wake times several days before departure can reduce circadian misalignment and minimize jet lag's effects. Avoiding screens before bedtime and managing competition anxiety through relaxation techniques can also improve sleep quality. Personalized medication approaches, guided by genetic testing, can help determine optimal timing and dosing of sleep aids when needed.

The science clearly shows that sleep represents a crucial factor in athletic success. Athletes who prioritize sleep by aiming for at least 8 h nightly typically perform better, recover faster, and face lower injury risks than their sleep-deprived counterparts [1]. This highlights that sleep quality is a key factor alongside physical training and nutrition in an athlete's preparation for competition. Modern sleep medicine increasingly focuses on personalized approaches, using genetic testing to understand how each athlete metabolizes sleep medications and adapting interventions accordingly.

Understanding sleep's role in athletic performance leads to better training approaches. Coaches increasingly recognize that pushing athletes through excessive training while sacrificing sleep can actually harm performance. Instead, building adequate rest periods into training schedules and monitoring sleep quality can help athletes reach their full potential while staying healthy. Advanced monitoring systems now provide real-time feedback on sleep quality and recovery status, while periodic melatonin assessments guide circadian phase alignment strategies allowing for truly personalized sleep optimization strategies that account for each athlete's unique biological characteristics.

The future of sleep optimization in athletics continues evolving with emerging technologies. Some professional sports teams now employ dedicated sleep specialists who work alongside strength coaches and nutritionists. These specialists analyze not just traditional sleep metrics but also examine how factors like training intensity, travel schedules, and competition timing affect individual athletes' sleep needs. This comprehensive approach helps create precisely tailored sleep strategies that adapt to each phase of an athlete's competitive season, from pre-season training through peak competition periods and into recovery phases.

References

1. Walsh NP, Halson SL, Sargent C, Roach GD, Nédélec M, Gupta L, Leeder J, Fullagar HH, Coutts AJ, Edwards BJ, Pullinger SA, Robertson CM, Burniston JG, Lastella M, Le Meur Y, Hausswirth C, Bender AM, Grandner MA, Samuels CH. Sleep and the athlete: narrative review and 2021 expert consensus recommendations. Br J Sports Med. 2020:bjsports-2020-102025 PMID: 33144349.
2. Montero A, Stevens D, Adams R, Drummond M. Sleep and mental health issues in current and former athletes: a mini review. Front Psychol. 2022;13:868614. PMID: 35465516.
3. Huang K, Ihm J. Sleep and injury risk. Curr Sports Med Rep. 2021;20(6):286–90. PMID: 34099605.
4. Vitale JA, Weydahl A. Chronotype, physical activity, and sport performance: a systematic review. Sports Med. 2017;47(9):1859–68. PMID: 28493061.
5. Cook JD, Charest J. Sleep and performance in professional athletes. Curr Sleep Med Rep. 2023;9(1):56–81. PMID: 36683842.
6. Zaffanello M, Pietrobelli A, Cavarzere P, Guzzo A, Antoniazzi F. Complex relationship between growth hormone and sleep in children: insights, discrepancies, and implications. Front Endocrinol (Lausanne). 2024;14:1332114. PMID: 38327902.
7. Carrard J, Rigort AC, Appenzeller-Herzog C, Colledge F, Königstein K, Hinrichs T, Schmidt-Trucksäss A. Diagnosing overtraining syndrome: a scoping review. Sports Health. 2022;14(5):665–73. PMID: 34496702.

Part III

The World of Sleep Disorders

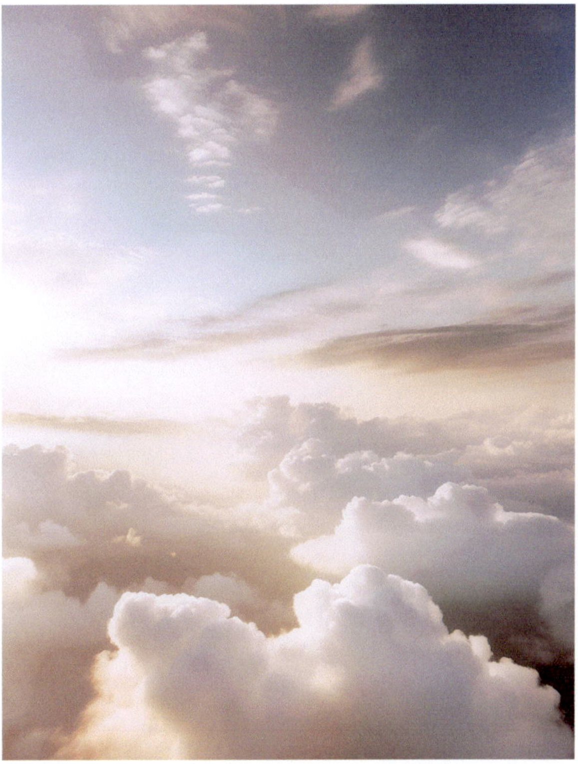

Fig. 1 Transitional 2. (Image generated using the prompt "Soft sunset clouds in sky; modern style illustration," by Adobe, Adobe Firefly, 2024. (https://firefly.adobe.com/))

The World of Sleep Disorders 19

19.1 Understanding Sleep Disorders: A Modern Health Challenge

Sleep disorders represent one of modern society's most significant yet often overlooked health challenges. While most people experience occasional sleep difficulties, true sleep or wakefulness disorders affect a staggering number of individuals—approximately 70 million adults in the United States alone, or approximately 1 in 3 adults [2]. Even more concerning, nearly half of all Americans report struggling with sleep at least weekly, suggesting that poor sleep has become a widespread public health issue [3].

The field of sleep medicine recognizes over 80 distinct sleep disorders, each with its own characteristics, causes, and treatment approaches [4]. These range from common conditions like insomnia, which makes it difficult to fall or stay asleep, to less familiar disorders like narcolepsy, which causes sudden, uncontrollable sleep attacks during the day. Some disorders, like sleep apnea, directly affect breathing during sleep, while others, such as restless legs syndrome, make it difficult to fall asleep due to uncomfortable sensations in the body. Sleep disorders are grouped into six major categories: insomnia disorders, sleep-related breathing disorders, central disorders of hypersomnolence, circadian rhythm sleep-wake disorders, parasomnias, and sleep-related movement disorders. This classification system helps clinicians diagnose and treat these conditions more effectively.

Sleep disorders affect nearly every aspect of health and daily function. During waking hours, people with sleep disorders often experience profound fatigue that goes beyond simple tiredness. This fatigue can impair judgment and reaction time to a degree comparable to alcohol intoxication—a finding that has serious implications for both personal and public safety. Many people with sleep disorders describe feeling as if they're moving through their day in a fog, struggling to concentrate or make decisions.

The physical health impact of sleep disorders proves particularly concerning [5]. Research has revealed strong connections between poor sleep and various chronic

A. Juginović, *Sleep Science Made Simple*,
https://doi.org/10.1007/978-3-031-92060-8_19

conditions. People with untreated sleep apnea face significantly higher risks of high blood pressure, heart disease, and stroke. Those with chronic insomnia show increased rates of diabetes and obesity. Even our immune system suffers when sleep becomes disrupted, making us more susceptible to infections and potentially slowing healing processes.

Mental health and sleep disorders share a complex, two-way relationship explained in one of the previous chapters in more detail [5]. Sleep disruption can trigger or worsen anxiety and depression, while these mental health conditions often make it harder to sleep well. This creates a challenging cycle that can be difficult to break without appropriate treatment. Recent research has revealed that this connection goes beyond mere correlation—sleep disruption actually changes how our brain processes emotional information, making us more vulnerable to stress and negative emotions.

The workplace impact of sleep disorders extends far beyond individual productivity. Sleep-deprived workers make more mistakes, have more accidents, and show increased rates of absenteeism [6]. In high-risk industries like transportation and healthcare, the consequences can be particularly severe. The estimated annual cost of fatigue-related workplace incidents reaches up to $400 billion in the United States alone, reflecting both direct medical costs and lost productivity [6].

Perhaps most alarming is the role of sleep disorders in public safety. Drowsy driving causes thousands of fatal accidents each year, with many more non-fatal crashes and near-misses going unreported. Shift workers, who often struggle with disrupted sleep patterns, face particularly high risks. Major industrial accidents, including nuclear power plant incidents and oil spills, have been linked to fatigue and sleep disruption among workers [1].

The good news is that most sleep disorders respond well to treatment when properly diagnosed. Modern sleep medicine offers various effective interventions, from behavioral techniques that help reset sleep patterns to advanced medical devices that maintain open airways during sleep. Some people benefit from medication, while others might need changes in their sleep environment or daily routines. The key lies in recognizing sleep disorders as serious medical conditions that require proper evaluation and treatment.

As we explore specific sleep disorders in the following chapters, we'll examine their unique characteristics, understand their causes, and discuss current treatment approaches. This knowledge proves essential not only for healthcare providers but for anyone seeking to understand and improve their sleep. With proper recognition and treatment of sleep disorders, we can work toward better sleep health for individuals and society as a whole.

References

1. Mitler MM, Carskadon MA, Czeisler CA, Dement WC, Dinges DF, Graeber RC. Catastrophes, sleep, and public policy: consensus report. Sleep. 1988;11(1):100–109. PMID: 3283909.
2. Institute of Medicine (US) Committee on Sleep Medicine and Research. Sleep disorders and sleep deprivation: an unmet public health problem. Colten HR, Altevogt BM, editors. Washington: National Academies Press (US); 2006. PMID: 20669438.

3. Di H, Guo Y, Daghlas I, Wang L, Liu G, Pan A, Liu L, Shan Z. Evaluation of sleep habits and disturbances among US adults, 2017-2020. JAMA Netw Open. 2022;5(11):e2240788. PMID: 36346632.
4. Thorpy MJ. Classification of sleep disorders. Neurotherapeutics. 2012;9(4):687–701. PMID: 22976557.
5. Institute of Medicine (US) Committee on Sleep Medicine and Research. Chapter 3: extent and health consequences of chronic sleep loss and sleep disorders. In: Colten HR, Altevogt BM, editors. Sleep disorders and sleep deprivation: an unmet public health problem. Washington (DC): National Academies Press (US); 2006. https://www.ncbi.nlm.nih.gov/books/NBK19961/.
6. Hafner M, Stepanek M, Taylor J, Troxel WM, van Stolk C. Why sleep matters-the economic costs of insufficient sleep: a cross-country comparative analysis. Rand Health Q. 2017;6(4):11. PMID: 28983434.

Customizing Sleep Treatments: A Targeted Approach to Health

20

20.1 Personalizing Sleep Treatment: Beyond One-Size-Fits-All

Modern sleep medicine increasingly recognizes that effective treatment requires individualized solutions. Just as we all have unique fingerprints, our sleep patterns, biological rhythms, and responses to treatment vary significantly. This understanding has led to more sophisticated, personalized approaches to treating sleep disorders.

At the heart of personalized sleep medicine is a key insight: genetic differences influence how individuals metabolize sleep medications [1]. Through pharmacogenomic testing, doctors can now determine how quickly or slowly a person metabolizes different sleep medications. Some people break down these medications rapidly, potentially needing higher doses to achieve proper effects, while others process them slowly, risking next-day grogginess from standard doses. This genetic insight helps doctors prescribe more precise dosages, reducing side effects while improving treatment effectiveness. While this approach may not always produce ideal outcomes, it remains a valuable tool in the clinician's arsenal.

Our internal biological clocks also vary significantly among individuals. Scientists can now assess when a person's body naturally begins producing melatonin (known as dim light melatonin onset or DLMO) to understand their unique circadian rhythm. This can even be used as a diagnostic tool to understand each individual's melatonin cycle which is a key indicator of your circadian rhythm. This knowledge is important for timing treatments effectively (e.g., knowing when to administer caffeine, bright light, or melatonin when traveling across time zones to minimize jet lag).

The causes of sleep disorders can differ dramatically between individuals, even when symptoms appear similar. Consider two individuals diagnosed with insomnia—one might struggle to sleep due to anxiety, while another's sleep problems stem from an irregular work schedule. These different root causes require different treatment approaches. The person with anxiety-related insomnia might benefit most

A. Juginovic, *Sleep Science Made Simple*,
https://doi.org/10.1007/978-3-031-92060-8_20

from cognitive behavioral therapy and stress management techniques, while the shift worker might need strategies to manage their circadian rhythm disruption.

Natural sleep timing preferences, often called chronotypes, simply refer to when your body naturally wants to sleep and wake. Some people are "morning people" (early birds or "larks") who naturally wake early and feel most alert in the morning, while "night owls" prefer to stay up late and sleep in. These patterns are partly genetic and reflect each person's underlying biological rhythm. Productivity, cognitive performance, and overall well-being improve when our daily schedules align with our natural chronotypes. Rather than fighting against these natural tendencies, adjusting work and activity schedules to match your chronotype can lead to better performance, reduced fatigue, and improved satisfaction compared to forcing everyone into the same rigid schedule. Of course, all of us understand that in some instances this is not possible.

Understanding individual differences has practical implications for treatment [1]. For example, a medication that benefits one person may be ineffective or cause side effects in another due to genetic differences in drug metabolism. Similarly, the ideal timing for light therapy or melatonin supplementation depends on a person's unique circadian rhythm. Even lifestyle recommendations require customization—exercise timing that suits a morning-oriented person may not work for a natural night owl.

Personalized approaches may also improve treatment outcomes—not only due to biological factors, but because patients feel more engaged when their therapy reflects their individual needs. When patients learn that their treatment plan considers their unique genetic makeup, circadian rhythm, and lifestyle factors, they are often more likely to adhere to the treatment plan.

The future of sleep medicine lies in increasingly sophisticated personalization. New technologies continue to emerge to assess individual sleep patterns, circadian rhythms, and genetic factors affecting sleep. These advances help doctors fine-tune treatments more precisely, leading to more effective solutions for sleep disorders. By recognizing and working with individual differences, modern sleep medicine can offer more effective, safer, and better-tailored solutions for the millions of people struggling with sleep disorders.

Reference

1. Garbarino S, Bragazzi NL. Revolutionizing sleep health: the emergence and impact of personalized sleep medicine. J Pers Med. 2024;14(6):598. PMID: 38929819.

Insomnia

21

21.1 Insomnia—The Most Prevalent Sleep Disorder

21.1.1 Understanding Insomnia: The Search for Sleep

We all know that frustrating feeling of lying awake at night, watching the minutes tick by. But while occasional sleepless nights are common, true insomnia involves a persistent struggle with sleep that significantly affects daily life. Think of insomnia like a car engine that won't shut off—even when you're physically and mentally exhausted, your brain keeps running, making sleep feel impossible. Insomnia often traps people in a frustrating cycle—the harder they try to sleep, the more elusive it becomes. Over time, this can lead to months or even years of disrupted rest.

Nearly a third of adults experience significant insomnia at some point in their lives, making it the most common sleep disorder [1, 2]. Remember how we discussed the complex interplay between your brain's sleep and wake systems? With insomnia, this delicate balance is disrupted. For some, it appears suddenly during times of stress—perhaps during a difficult period at work or while going through personal challenges. The stress response system becomes over active, making it difficult to transition into sleep. For others, insomnia develops gradually, starting with a few bad nights that eventually snowball into a chronic condition that can last months or years.

Insomnia manifests in different ways depending on the individual. Some people lie awake for hours, their minds racing despite physical exhaustion—this difficulty falling asleep is called sleep onset insomnia. Others fall asleep quickly but wake repeatedly throughout the night (sleep maintenance insomnia), watching the clock as minutes crawl by. Still others experience early morning awakening insomnia, finding themselves alert at 3 AM when their brain's wake-promoting circuits activate too early, unable to return to sleep. What unites these experiences is the profound effect on daily life—the persistent fatigue, difficulty concentrating, and emotional strain that follow disrupted sleep.

A. Juginović, *Sleep Science Made Simple*,
https://doi.org/10.1007/978-3-031-92060-8_21

The causes of insomnia often reads like a catalog of modern stressors [1]. Stress from work or personal life tops the list as the most common trigger—your brain's stress response system stays activated, making it difficult to transition into sleep. Poor sleep habits play a major role too, especially irregular sleep schedules or excessive screen time before bed that confuse your brain's natural sleep-wake rhythms. Lifestyle factors like evening caffeine consumption, late-night eating, or lack of regular exercise can all contribute. Sometimes, environmental factors are to blame—a bedroom that's too warm, too noisy, or too bright can prevent your brain from properly transitioning to sleep. Travel across time zones (jet lag) or shift work can severely disrupt your circadian rhythms, leading to insomnia. For women, hormonal changes during menstruation, pregnancy, or menopause often trigger sleep problems. What makes insomnia particularly challenging is that these factors often combine and reinforce each other—for instance, stress might lead to poor sleep habits, which then create more stress about sleep.

The duration of insomnia varies significantly, and understanding these patterns helps determine both its severity and treatment approach [1]. Acute insomnia, lasting a few days to a few weeks, often resolves on its own once the triggering event (like a stressful work deadline or jet lag) passes. However, for about 20% of people, acute insomnia transitions into chronic insomnia, defined as sleep difficulties occurring at least three times per week for 3 months or longer [3]. Some people experience episodic insomnia, where periods of normal sleep alternate with weeks or months of poor sleep, often triggered by recurring stressors or seasonal changes. Without proper treatment, chronic insomnia can persist for years, with some people struggling for a decade or more (Fig. 21.1). The longer insomnia continues, the more likely it is to develop its own self-perpetuating cycle—sleep difficulties lead to anxiety about sleep, which then makes sleep even harder to achieve.

Primary insomnia occurs on its own, not caused by other health conditions or medications. It's as if the brain gets stuck in an 'on' position, with overactive wake-promoting circuits unable to shift into sleep mode even when tired. Some people may be more biologically predisposed to this type of insomnia, perhaps due to an overactive stress response system or genetic factors that make their sleep-wake regulation more vulnerable to disruption.

Secondary insomnia, more common but no less challenging, develops alongside other conditions [1]. Chronic pain can make finding a comfortable sleeping position difficult, as pain signals keep wake-promoting circuits active. Depression and anxiety can fill nights with worried thoughts that prevent sleep by increasing activity in brain regions involved in emotional processing and arousal. Even certain medications (e.g., antidepressants), while treating one condition, might inadvertently disrupt sleep patterns by affecting neurotransmitters involved in sleep regulation. Distinguishing between primary and secondary insomnia is essential for tailoring effective treatment strategies, as each type might require different approaches.

The impact of chronic insomnia extends far beyond tired mornings. During the day, individuals with chronic insomnia often describe feeling mentally foggy, struggling to concentrate or remember simple things. This happens because sleep deprivation affects the prefrontal cortex—your brain's command center for

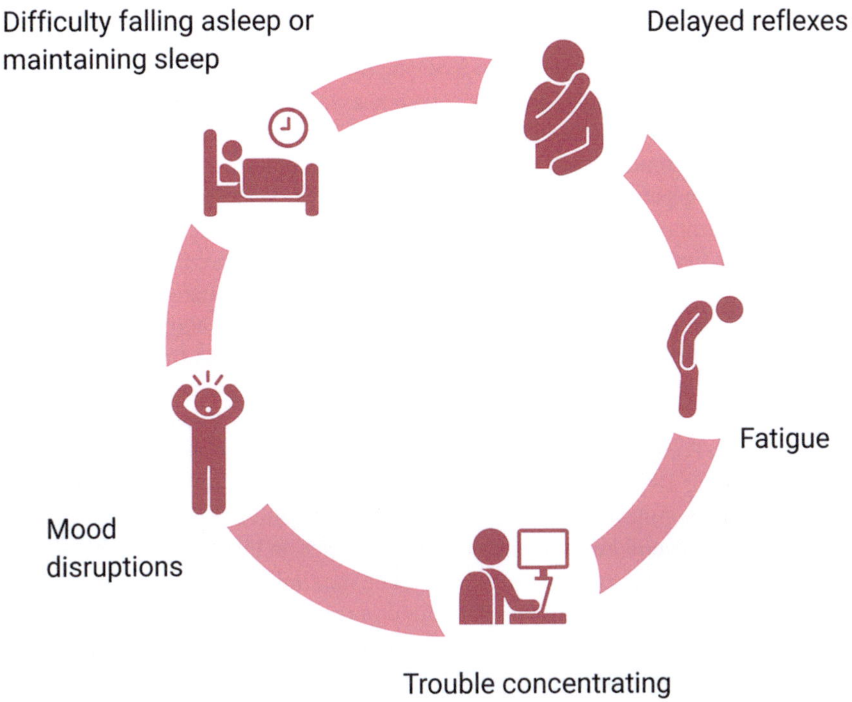

Fig. 21.1 Illustration showing the key symptoms of insomnia. ("Image generated by ChatGPT (OpenAI), 2025. Used with permission")

complex thinking and decision-making. Work performance suffers, relationships become strained, and even basic tasks feel more challenging. The brain, deprived of proper sleep, becomes less efficient at processing emotions, making people more vulnerable to stress and mood changes. Chronic insomnia has also been linked to long-term health risks, including elevated rates of depression, anxiety, and cardiovascular disease, highlighting why proper treatment is so crucial.

21.1.2 Diagnosing and Treating Insomnia

Diagnosing insomnia requires careful work because sleep problems often intertwine with other aspects of health and daily life [1]. Sleep specialists typically begin by taking a full history of someone's sleep difficulties—not just current symptoms, but how sleep patterns have changed over time. A thorough evaluation includes reviewing medical history, medications, lifestyle habits, and mental health. Keeping a sleep diary for one to several weeks often reveals important patterns that people might not notice otherwise. Patients complete these simple yet informative diaries and track not only sleep times but also factors like caffeine and medication intake, exercise, stress levels, and even room temperature. These detailed records can show, for instance, how a late-afternoon coffee might affect sleep quality, or how different bedtime routines influence how quickly someone falls asleep.

Sometimes, especially when the cause remains unclear or symptoms suggest other disorders, doctors recommend a sleep study using polysomnography. While not always necessary for diagnosing insomnia, these overnight studies can help rule out other sleep disorders that might masquerade as insomnia. For instance, someone might think they have insomnia when actually sleep apnea disrupts their rest, or restless legs syndrome prevents them from falling asleep. The study monitors brain waves, breathing patterns, heart rate, and body movements throughout the night, providing a comprehensive picture of sleep architecture. This can reveal whether someone truly lies awake for hours, as they perceive, or whether they actually sleep more than they realize—a common phenomenon called sleep state misperception.

Effective insomnia treatment often requires a multi-component approach, with cognitive-behavioral therapy for insomnia (CBT-I) emerging as the most effective long-term treatment [4]. This specialized therapy typically spans 6–8 sessions and helps people identify and change unhelpful thoughts and behaviors that interfere with sleep [5]. For instance, someone might learn to recognize and challenge catastrophic thinking about sleep ("I'll never fall asleep" or "I can't function without 8 hours"), or develop new routines that help their body and mind prepare for sleep. CBT-I includes several key components: sleep restriction therapy (temporarily limiting time in bed to increase sleep efficiency, i.e., maximizing the proportion of time in bed that is actually spent asleep), stimulus control (which aims to strengthen your mental association of the bed with sleep), relaxation techniques, and education about sleep hygiene. Research shows CBT-I improves both sleep quality and long-term treatment outcomes [1].

Before turning to medication, treatment should begin with improving sleep habits and the sleep environment—what sleep specialists call "sleep hygiene." This means creating conditions that promote natural sleep by working with your brain's sleep-wake circuits. Keeping consistent sleep schedules helps maintain proper circadian rhythm, while managing evening light exposure (especially the blue light from screens) supports your brain's natural melatonin production. Even small behavioral adjustments can meaningfully improve sleep: maintaining a cool bedroom temperature (around 18 °C/65 °F) supports the natural drop in core body temperature that helps initiate sleep; creating a dark, quiet environment reduces arousal-promoting sensory input to your brain; and developing relaxing bedtime routines signals to your brain that it's time to transition to sleep mode.

Many people find additional relief through complementary approaches that help calm an overactive nervous system [1]. Mindfulness meditation can help break the cycle of anxious thoughts about sleep by teaching individuals to observe their thoughts without getting caught up in them. Progressive muscle relaxation, which involves systematically tensing and then releasing different muscle groups throughout the body, reduces physical tension that might interfere with sleep onset. The 4–7-8 breathing technique, where you inhale for 4 s, hold for 7 s, and exhale for 8 s, helps activate the parasympathetic nervous system to promote relaxation. Gentle evening yoga can help transition your body from the sympathetic ("fight or flight") to parasympathetic ("rest and digest") state. Some people also benefit from chronotherapy—strategically timing exposure to light and darkness to reset disrupted circadian rhythms. Addressing specific lifestyle factors proves crucial too: limiting caffeine to the morning hours (remember its 4–7-h half-life), finishing exercise to end at least 2–3 h before bedtime, and finding ways to manage irregular work schedules can all contribute to better sleep.

Sleep medications can provide temporary relief, but they require careful medical oversight [1]. While these medications can help break acute insomnia cycles, they don't address the underlying causes of chronic sleep problems. For insomnia treatment, we have several major medication classes: benzodiazepines (like temazepam and triazolam), non-benzodiazepine receptor agonists or "Z-drugs"(like zolpidem, eszopiclone, and zaleplon), melatonin receptor agonists (like ramelteon), orexin receptor antagonists (such as suvorexant and daridorexant), and certain antidepressants used at low doses (such as doxepin). Each works through distinct neural pathways—benzodiazepines and Z-drugs enhance the inhibitory effects of the neurotransmitter GABA, melatonin agonists mimic the body's natural sleep hormone, orexin antagonists block wake-promoting signals, and low-dose doxepin primarily blocks histamine receptors that cause wakefulness. For different insomnia types, medication selection varies based on properties like half-life and action timing. Sleep-onset insomnia typically responds to shorter-acting medications that work quickly (like zaleplon, zolpidem, triazolam, or ramelteon). Sleep maintenance insomnia benefits from medications with longer duration (like eszopiclone, temazepam, suvorexant, or doxepin) that help prevent nighttime awakenings. Combined insomnia (disrupted sleep onset and maintenance) may require medications that address both problems. Over-the-counter options like diphenhydramine, melatonin, and herbal supplements (valerian, tryptophan) have limited evidence supporting their long-term effectiveness. Certain prescription drugs may lead to dependency and alter sleep architecture, particularly with long-term use [1]. This explains why sleep specialists typically recommend cognitive behavioral therapy for insomnia (CBT-I) as the first-line treatment, with medications used cautiously for short periods while developing longer-term behavioral solutions. The key lies in finding a sustainable approach that addresses both the symptoms and underlying causes of insomnia.

Recovery from chronic insomnia often takes time and patience, similar to rehabilitation after an injury. Some people find relief quickly once they identify and address specific triggers—perhaps changing their work schedule or improving their sleep environment. Others need to try various approaches before finding their path to better sleep. The process might involve setbacks and adjustments, but understanding this as normal helps prevent discouragement. The key lies in recognizing that improving sleep usually requires consistent effort, time, and usually professional guidance. Lasting improvement often requires a combined approach: integrating CBT-I with lifestyle changes and addressing coexisting health factors.

Left untreated, chronic insomnia can lead to serious health consequences that extend far beyond daytime fatigue [6]. Sleep deprivation disrupts biological systems across multiple levels. The immune system becomes less effective at fighting off infections, while inflammation throughout the body increases. Individuals with persistent insomnia develop higher levels of inflammatory markers, creating a state of chronic low-grade inflammation. Hormonal imbalances disrupt appetite regulation, increasing hunger and reducing satiety, which can contribute to weight gain and metabolic dysfunction. Ongoing sleep loss also reduces insulin sensitivity, often leading to glucose intolerance and raising the risk of type 2 diabetes. The risk of developing high blood pressure and heart disease rises substantially with ongoing sleep problems. Perhaps most concerning, chronic sleep disruption appears to affect brain health—increasing risks of anxiety, depression, and accelerated cognitive decline. Poor sleep quality correlates with increased deposits of proteins associated with neurodegenerative diseases, while consistently shortened sleep impairs the brain's ability to clear metabolic waste. This cascade of effects explains why addressing insomnia timely and effectively is crucial for overall health, as even modest improvements in sleep quality can significantly reduce these multisystem health risks.

Insomnia represents far more than just difficult nights—it's a complex condition that impacts nearly every aspect of health and well-being. From racing thoughts preventing sleep onset to frustrating early morning awakenings, insomnia manifests differently across individuals but consistently reduces quality of life. The condition's causes span from psychological factors like stress and anxiety to physiological issues and poor sleep habits. While chronic insomnia can lead to serious health consequences affecting everything from heart function to brain health, effective treatments exist. Through evidence-based approaches like cognitive behavioral therapy, lifestyle modifications, and carefully managed medication when necessary, patients can target both the symptoms and underlying causes of this widespread condition.

References

1. Naha S, Sivaraman M, Sahota P. Insomnia: a current review. Mo Med. 2024;121(1):44–51. PMID: 38404423; PMCID: PMC10887463.
2. Bhaskar S, Hemavathy D, Prasad S. Prevalence of chronic insomnia in adult patients and its correlation with medical comorbidities. J Family Med Prim Care. 2016;5(4):780–4. PMID: 28348990.
3. Penn Medicine News. 1 in 4 Americans develop insomnia each year [Internet]. Philadelphia: University of Pennsylvania Health System; 2018. Cited 2024 Dec 26. https://www.pennmedicine.org/news/news-releases/2018/june/1-in-4-americans-develop-insomnia-each-year
4. The Insomnia and Sleep Institute of Arizona. How effective is CBT-I for treating insomnia? [Internet]. Phoenix: The Insomnia and Sleep Institute of Arizona; Cited 2024 Jan 26. https://sleeplessinarizona.com/how-effective-is-cbt-i-for-treating-insomnia
5. Rossman J. Cognitive-behavioral therapy for insomnia: an effective and underutilized treatment for insomnia. Am J Lifestyle Med. 2019;13(6):544–7. PMID: 31662718.
6. Institute of Medicine (US) Committee on Sleep Medicine and Research. Chapter:3 extent and health consequences of chronic sleep loss and sleep disorders. In: Colten HR, Altevogt BM, editors. Sleep disorders and sleep deprivation: an unmet public health problem. Washington: National Academies Press (US); 2006. https://www.ncbi.nlm.nih.gov/books/NBK19961/.

Sleep Apnea 22

22.1 Sleep Apnea—When Breathing Stops

22.1.1 Sleep Apnea: An Introduction

Sleep apnea is a common and serious sleep disorder in which breathing repeatedly stops and starts during sleep. While essentially all of us experience brief pauses in breathing during sleep, people with sleep apnea face interruptions at least 5 times per hour on average during their sleep. These pauses (which manifest as reductions in airflow by at least 90%) last 10 s or longer and cause oxygen levels in the blood to drop by at least 3% [1]. These breathing disruptions can occur hundreds of times each night, often without the person being aware of them. If untreated, sleep apnea can increase the risk of a whole array of disorders that we will explore shortly.

The condition takes three main forms, each with distinct characteristics [1]. Obstructive Sleep Apnea (OSA), the most common type, occurs commonly when throat muscles relax too much during sleep, blocking the airway (Fig. 22.1). Think of it like a garden hose being stepped on—the flow stops because of physical blockage, even though the water pressure remains. Central Sleep Apnea (CSA), much less common but equally serious, happens when the brain fails to send proper breathing signals during sleep—like forgetting to turn the water on in our garden hose analogy. Some people experience Complex Sleep Apnea Syndrome (CompSAS), a form of sleep-disordered breathing in which central apneas persist or emerge when obstructive events are treated with positive airway pressure therapy.

A related condition called hypopnea represents periods of shallow breathing rather than complete stops [2]. During hypopnea episodes, breathing reduces by at least 30% for 10 s or more, leading to drops in blood oxygen levels. While not as dramatic as complete breathing stops, these episodes can also be disruptive to sleep quality and long-term health.

A. Juginović, *Sleep Science Made Simple*,
https://doi.org/10.1007/978-3-031-92060-8_22

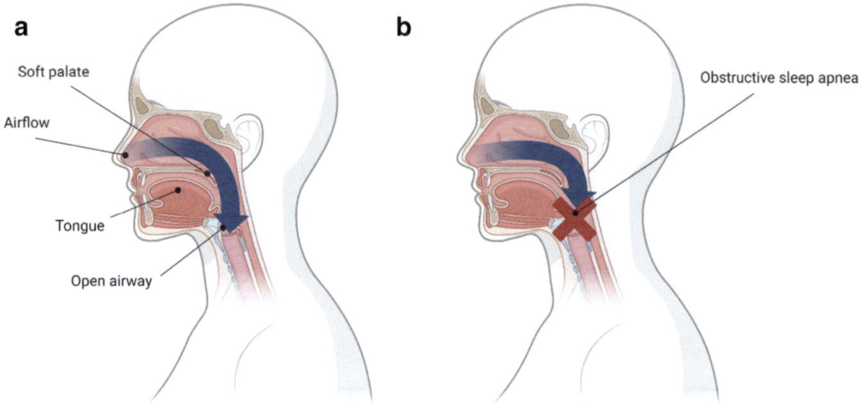

Fig. 22.1 Obstructive sleep apnea (**a**—Physiological state, **b**—Obstructive sleep apnea). ("Created in BioRender. Juginovic, A. (2025) https://BioRender.com/i01r459")

22.1.2 Understanding Sleep Apnea's Reach: Risk Factors and Prevalence

Sleep apnea is more prevalent than many people realize. Recent research suggests that between 9% and 38% of adults have some form of sleep apnea, with at least 25 million Americans affected [1]. These numbers continue rising, partly due to increasing obesity rates and our aging population.

Several factors increase sleep apnea risk, creating a complex web of genetic, anatomical, and lifestyle influences [3]. Weight plays a crucial role—people with a body mass index (BMI) over 25 face significantly higher risks, as excess tissue can compress their airways during sleep [4]. Neck size matters too, with risks increasing for men whose necks measure more than 43 cm (17 inches) around and women with necks larger than 38 cm (15 inches) [3, 5].

Gender influences sleep apnea risk in interesting ways [3]. Men generally face higher risks than women, but this difference narrows after menopause. Age also plays a significant role, with risk increasing notably after 40, though sleep apnea can affect people of any age, including children. Children face unique risk factors—enlarged tonsils and adenoids are actually the leading cause of sleep apnea in children, unlike adults where obesity often plays the primary role. When these lymphoid tissues become too large relative to the child's airway, they can obstruct breathing during sleep, leading to sleep apnea that may impair a child's growth, behavior, and cognitive development.

Anatomical features contribute to sleep apnea risk in ways that might surprise many people [3]. A narrow throat, large tongue, or small jaw can all increase the likelihood of airway collapse during sleep. Even nasal structure plays a role—a deviated septum or chronic nasal congestion can force mouth breathing during sleep, increasing the risk of apnea episodes. Family history significantly influences sleep apnea risk, suggesting genetic factors play an important role. If you have close relatives with sleep apnea, your own risk increases, though lifestyle choices can still greatly affect whether you develop the condition.

Certain lifestyle factors can either increase risk or worsen existing sleep apnea [3]. Alcohol consumption, especially in the evening, relaxes upper airway muscles and can increase the likelihood of breathing pauses. Smoking irritates and inflames the airways, potentially making them more prone to collapse during sleep. Even sleep position matters—sleeping on your back often makes sleep apnea worse because gravity pulls the tongue and soft tissues backward.

Understanding these risk factors helps both prevention and treatment. While we can't change our genetics or basic anatomy, many modifiable risk factors remain under our control. Maintaining a healthy weight, avoiding alcohol before bedtime, and treating nasal problems can significantly reduce sleep apnea risk or improve existing symptoms. For those already diagnosed with sleep apnea, understanding these risk factors helps explain why certain lifestyle changes form an important part of treatment alongside medical interventions.

Recent research continues revealing new aspects of sleep apnea risk [3]. Scientists have identified specific genetic markers associated with sleep apnea risk, opening possibilities for earlier identification of high-risk individuals. Studies also show that certain medical conditions, including type 2 diabetes and heart failure, share complex relationships with sleep apnea, each potentially worsening the other.

22.1.3 Different Types of Sleep Apnea

22.1.3.1 Obstructive Sleep Apnea: When Airways Collapse

Obstructive Sleep Apnea (OSA) is the most common form of sleep apnea, caused by repeated collapse of the upper airway during sleep [3]. Think of the airway like a flexible tube—when the muscles supporting it relax too much during sleep, the tube can collapse, either partially or completely blocking airflow. These collapses typically happen at specific points in the throat, particularly where the soft palate meets the back of the throat or where the tongue falls backward and blocks the airway.

During these episodes, which can last from several seconds to over a minute, the body continues trying to breathe. The chest and diaphragm muscles work harder and harder, but like trying to drink through a pinched straw, these efforts are ineffective. This struggle for breath often leads to drops in blood oxygen levels, triggering brief awakenings that fragment sleep throughout the night.

The symptoms of OSA range from dramatic to subtle. While loud snoring often serves as the most noticeable sign, many people with OSA experience morning headaches, excessive daytime sleepiness, and difficulty concentrating. Some wake up gasping or feeling like they're choking, while others might not remember waking at all, despite their sleep being frequently disrupted. The snoring occurs because the partially collapsed airway creates turbulent airflow, causing soft tissues to vibrate—though not all individuals who snore have sleep apnea.

A particularly serious condition that can coexist with OSA in people with severe obesity is obesity hypoventilation syndrome (OHS), also referred to as Pickwickian syndrome [6]. In OHS, excess weight in the chest and abdomen impairs breathing, leading to inadequate ventilation even during wakefulness. When combined with obstructive sleep apnea, this can result in dangerously low oxygen levels and elevated carbon dioxide in the blood, increasing the risk of heart failure if left untreated.

22.1.3.2 Central Sleep Apnea: When the Brain's Signals Fail

Unlike OSA, Central Sleep Apnea (CSA) arises from a communication problem between the brain and breathing muscles [7]. During normal breathing, the brain constantly monitors oxygen and carbon dioxide levels, adjusting breathing rate and depth accordingly. In CSA, this careful control system malfunctions, resulting in episodes where the brain fails to transmit appropriate signals to initiate breathing.

CSA can arise from various medical conditions affecting the central nervous system [7]. Neurological conditions like Parkinson's disease or stroke can disrupt the brain's breathing control centers. Heart failure can trigger a form of CSA through complex mechanisms involving blood flow and oxygen sensing. Certain medications, particularly opioids, can also disrupt central respiratory regulation.

The symptoms of CSA often differ subtly from those of OSA. While both conditions can cause daytime sleepiness and poor sleep quality, people with CSA typically don't snore as loudly as those with OSA. Instead, they might experience more pronounced shortness of breath or difficulty falling asleep. Some people with CSA report a distinctive pattern where they awaken with a sensation of breathlessness, as if they had forgotten to breathe.

22.1.3.3 Central Sleep Apnea with Cheyne-Stokes Respiration: A Distinctive Breathing Pattern

One particularly fascinating form of CSA involves a unique breathing pattern called central sleep apnea with Cheyne-Stokes breathing [8]. Unlike typical central sleep apnea where breathing stops and restarts, this pattern looks more like ocean waves—breathing gradually gets deeper and deeper, then becomes progressively shallower until it stops completely. Each cycle, lasting 60–90 s, repeats throughout sleep, creating a pattern of recurring apneas (breathing pauses) that disrupts sleep in a very distinct way.

This unusual breathing pattern often appears in people with heart failure, where it can affect up to 50% of patients [9]. To understand why, imagine your body's breathing control system as a thermostat adjusting room temperature. Normally, your brain receives quick updates about oxygen and carbon dioxide levels in your blood and adjusts breathing accordingly. However, in heart failure, blood moves more slowly through the body. By the time blood carrying information about oxygen and carbon dioxide levels reaches the brain's breathing control centers, the information is outdated. It's like trying to adjust your room temperature with a thermostat that's getting readings from 15 min ago—you'll constantly over-correct, making the room too hot, then too cold, in a continuous cycle. In the same way, your brain's breathing adjustments consistently overshoot or undershoot what your body actually needs, leading to this wave-like pattern of breathing followed by apneas.

High altitude can trigger a similar breathing pattern, even in otherwise healthy people [9]. Above about 2500 m (8000 feet), the thinner air leads to a condition called high-altitude periodic breathing. Just as your heart failure patients' brains overcompensate for delayed signals, your brain at high altitude overcompensates for lower oxygen levels by triggering deeper breathing. This overcompensation leads to a drop in carbon dioxide levels that temporarily halts breathing—another type of central sleep apnea. This explains why some mountain climbers experience disrupted sleep until they acclimatize to the altitude, as their bodies learn to fine-tune this respiratory control system to work efficiently with less oxygen.

22.1.3.4 Complex Sleep Apnea Syndrome: When Problems Combine

Complex sleep apnea syndrome (CompSAS) is the term used to describe a form of sleep-disordered breathing in which repeated central apneas (>5/h) persist or emerge when obstructive events are treated with positive airway pressure therapy, a treatment that uses air pressure to keep the airway open through a device that one uses only when sleeping (e.g., CPAP machine—Continuous Positive Airway Pressure) [10]. Unlike simple obstructive or central sleep apnea, CompSAS develops when patients who primarily have obstructive sleep apnea suddenly exhibit central apneas during treatment. Think of it as your respiratory system facing a paradoxical challenge—the therapy that successfully opens your airway (addressing the obstructive component) somehow triggers your brain to temporarily stop sending proper breathing signals (creating a central component).

The underlying mechanisms of CompSAS involve a delicate balance in breathing regulation [10]. When CPAP successfully opens the airway, it can sometimes make breathing too efficient, washing out too much carbon dioxide from the blood. This drop in carbon dioxide can trick the brain into thinking it doesn't need to breathe, causing temporary breathing pauses. Additionally, the pressure from CPAP therapy can trigger certain receptors in the lungs and airways that affect breathing patterns. This creates a frustrating cycle where fixing one problem (airway obstruction) inadvertently creates another (central apneas), leading to disrupted sleep despite treatment. This type of apnea is relatively common, affecting up to 15% of the sleep apnea population [10].

Treatment for CompSAS requires careful monitoring and a personalized approach. In most patients (about 75–80%), the central apnea component resolves on its own after continued CPAP use over a period of weeks to months [10]. It's as if the brain's breathing control center needs time to recalibrate once the obstruction is resolved. For those with persistent central apneas despite CPAP therapy, more advanced respiratory assist devices may be necessary. More advanced devices like bilevel therapy (BiPAP, which uses two different pressure levels—higher when breathing in and lower when breathing out to help you breathe more easily versus CPAP which provides continuous pressure). Even more refined ventilatory support comes from adaptive servo-ventilation (ASV), which can adjust pressure support breath by breath to match the patient's changing needs. ASV works like a more intelligent CPAP, anticipating each breath and providing just the right amount of support. However, it's important to note that ASV isn't suitable for everyone—particularly some patients with severe heart failure, where it might actually be harmful. This highlights why proper evaluation and monitoring by sleep specialists remains crucial for effective treatment.

22.1.4 Diagnosing and Treating Sleep Apnea

Unless you have a bed partner who notices pauses in your breathing during sleep, sleep apnea is often difficult to recognize without external input. You might experience symptoms like persistent daytime sleepiness (even after what feels like a full night's sleep), morning headaches, difficulty concentrating, or irritability, but these are also seen in other sleep disorders [3]. Some people wake up gasping or with a dry mouth, while others experience unexplained fatigue or high blood pressure. If you snore loudly and frequently, especially with noticeable pauses in breathing that your bed partner might observe, these could be important clues. Because these symptoms arise during sleep, identifying them often requires observation by others or professional testing.

The path to diagnosing sleep apnea begins in a specialized sleep laboratory, where sophisticated monitoring equipment reveals what happens during sleep [3]. During this overnight study, called polysomnography, trained technicians track brain activity, heart rate, breathing effort, airflow, and oxygen saturation. Think of it as creating a detailed map of your night's sleep, tracking everything from brain waves and heart rhythm to breathing patterns and oxygen levels.

This comprehensive overnight monitoring serves as the gold standard for diagnosing sleep apnea. The equipment can detect breathing pauses as brief as 10 s and drops in blood oxygen levels as small as 3%. More importantly, it helps distinguish between different types of sleep apnea by monitoring muscle activity. When someone has obstructive sleep apnea, the monitoring shows their breathing muscles (chest and abdomen) working hard against a blocked airway. In central sleep apnea, these same muscles remain quiet, indicating the brain isn't sending proper breathing signals.

Sleep apnea severity is quantified using the Apnea-Hypopnea Index (AHI), which counts how many breathing pauses occur each hour during sleep [3]. Someone with mild sleep apnea might experience 5–15 interruptions per hour, while severe cases can involve 30 or more episodes. A related measure, the Respiratory Disturbance Index (RDI), also includes more subtle breathing irregularities—such as respiratory effort-related arousals (RERAs)—which briefly disrupt sleep without meeting the criteria for full apneas or hypopneas.

Before recommending a full sleep study, doctors often begin with screening tools to assess sleep apnea risk [3]. These questionnaires explore factors like snoring patterns, daytime sleepiness, and observed breathing pauses. Commonly used examples include the STOP-Bang questionnaire, which evaluates Snoring, Tiredness, Observed apneas, high blood Pressure, Body mass index, Age, Neck circumference, and Gender, and the Epworth Sleepiness Scale, which measures daytime sleepiness by asking individuals to rate their likelihood of dozing off in different everyday situations. Another frequently used tool is the Pittsburgh Sleep Quality Index (PSQI), a broader questionnaire that assesses overall sleep quality and disturbances over the past month, including factors like sleep duration, latency (time needed to fall asleep), and perceived sleep efficiency (the percentage of time spent asleep relative to the total time spent in bed).

While home sleep tests offer a more convenient alternative to laboratory studies, they provide less detailed information. These devices focus primarily on breathing patterns and oxygen levels, missing the rich data about brain activity and muscle movement that laboratory studies capture (e.g., polysomnography). However, they can prove appropriate for some patients, particularly those showing clear signs of moderate to severe sleep apnea without other complicating medical conditions. Once sleep apnea is diagnosed, whether through home testing or laboratory studies, treatment can begin—and the treatment landscape has transformed significantly in recent years.

Sleep apnea treatment has evolved dramatically in recent years, moving from one-size-fits-all approaches to carefully tailored solutions that match each person's specific breathing patterns and lifestyle needs. While we can't typically cure sleep apnea, modern medicine offers numerous effective ways to manage the condition and significantly improve both sleep quality and overall health.

The cornerstone of sleep apnea treatment remains CPAP (Continuous Positive Airway Pressure) therapy, which acts like an invisible splint keeping the airway open throughout the night [3]. The device delivers a gentle stream of pressurized air (typically between 5 and 15 cm H_2O) through a mask worn during sleep. (Fig. 22.2). While some people initially find the mask challenging to use, modern CPAP technology has evolved significantly to address these concerns. Basic CPAP machines deliver a single, fixed pressure determined during your sleep study, but more advanced devices called APAP (Automatic Positive Airway Pressure) can automatically adjust pressure levels throughout the night based on your breathing patterns. All these machines come with masks in different styles and sizes to suit different preferences—from minimal designs that cover just the nose to fuller masks for those who breathe through their mouths during sleep.

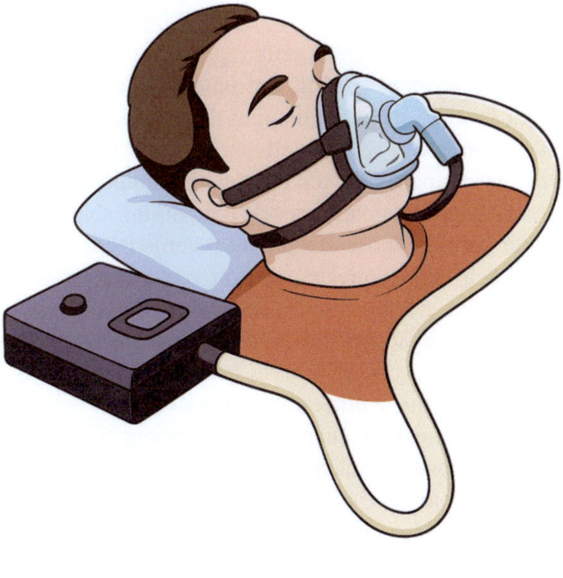

Fig. 22.2 CPAP therapy: continuous airflow support for sleep apnea treatment. ("Image generated by ChatGPT (OpenAI), 2025. Used with permission")

For those who find standard CPAP challenging, alternative devices offer more sophisticated solutions. BiPAP (Bi-level Positive Airway Pressure) machines provide two different pressure levels—one for breathing in and another for breathing out—making it easier to exhale against the airflow. Even more advanced, adaptive servo-ventilation (ASV) adjusts pressure in real time, tailoring support to each breath—especially useful for central or complex sleep apnea.

Dental devices provide another valuable treatment option, particularly for mild to moderate cases or for people who can't tolerate CPAP. These specially designed oral appliances, made by dentists with expertise in sleep medicine, help position the jaw and tongue to keep the airway more open during sleep. They work particularly well for people whose sleep apnea worsens when sleeping on their back.

Weight management plays a pivotal role in treating sleep apnea, particularly since up to 45% of adults with obesity have obstructive sleep apnea (OSA) [11]. Even a modest 10–16% reduction in body weight can significantly reduce AHI by 30–50% and sometimes even cure mild cases of sleep apnea [12]. However, this creates a challenging cycle—poor sleep disrupts hormones that control appetite and metabolism, making weight loss more difficult, while excess weight worsens sleep apnea by adding pressure on the airway and affecting breathing control. Recent medical advances have opened new possibilities for addressing this connection. A new class of medications called GLP-1 receptor agonists (which mimic a natural hormone that helps control appetite and blood sugar, helping patients feel fuller and lose weight) show promising results in treating sleep apnea [13]. These medications help people feel fuller longer and crave less food, leading to significant weight loss. Not only do they help with weight loss, but they may also improve sleep apnea symptoms even before significant weight loss occurs, possibly through effects on upper airway muscle control and breathing regulation. This understanding has led to more integrated treatment approaches that address both sleep and weight management together, often combining CPAP therapy with weight management strategies for optimal results.

Some fascinating alternative approaches have shown promise in research studies. Breathing exercises using instruments like the didgeridoo can help reduce sleep apnea severity by strengthening the muscles that keep airways open during sleep [14]. More recently, innovative treatments like hypoglossal nerve stimulation have emerged, using implanted devices to stimulate the nerve controlling tongue movement and help maintain muscle tone during sleep [15].

For people whose sleep apnea stems from anatomical issues, surgical options might help. Procedures range from removing excess throat tissue (uvulopalatopharyngoplasty, which removes excess throat tissue to widen the airway) to repairing a deviated nasal septum or repositioning the jaw for better airway alignment [16]. While surgery typically serves as a last resort, it can either serve as primary treatment or help make other treatments like CPAP more effective.

Simple lifestyle changes complement all forms of sleep apnea treatment. Sleeping position matters significantly—side sleeping often reduces breathing problems compared to back sleeping [17]. Some people find success with creative solutions like sewing a tennis ball into the back of their pajamas to discourage back sleeping, while others benefit from specialized positioning pillows. Avoiding alcohol before bedtime and maintaining regular sleep schedules also help reduce breathing problems during sleep.

The key to successful treatment lies in understanding that no single approach works for everyone. Some people might need to try several treatments before finding their optimal solution, while others benefit from combining different approaches. Regular follow-up with sleep specialists helps ensure treatments remain effective and can be adjusted as needed to maintain good sleep quality.

22.1.5 The Long-Term Impact of Untreated Sleep Apnea

When sleep apnea goes untreated, it can trigger a cascade of health problems that extend far beyond poor sleep [18]. The repeated cycles of breathing interruption during sleep create a ripple effect throughout the body, affecting everything from heart health to brain function. Each pause in breathing briefly awakens your brain, sometimes hundreds of times per night, preventing you from getting the deep, restorative sleep your body needs. This fragmented sleep leads to more than just feeling tired—people often experience persistent mental fog, difficulty concentrating, memory problems, and mood changes including irritability and depression. Many describe feeling exhausted even after what seems like a full night's sleep, and some find themselves dozing off during everyday activities like reading or watching TV.

One of the most immediate and dangerous consequences of untreated sleep apnea appears on the road [18]. The chronic sleepiness caused by sleep apnea significantly increases accident risk, particularly for professional drivers. Studies show that drivers with untreated sleep apnea face up to five times higher risk of traffic accidents. Many people with untreated sleep apnea struggle to maintain attention while driving, experience slower reaction times, and might even experience brief "micro-sleeps"—brief, involuntary lapses in consciousness that can be deadly behind the wheel. This cognitive impairment becomes especially concerning when considering truck drivers or others operating heavy machinery, where a moment's lapse in attention can have devastating consequences.

The impact on the cardiovascular system is particularly concerning [18]. Each time breathing stops during sleep, oxygen levels in the blood drop, triggering a stress response in the body through the sympathetic nerve system. The heart must work harder, blood pressure rises, and blood vessels constrict. When this pattern repeats night after night—sometimes hundreds of times—it can lead to chronic high blood pressure and significantly increase the risk of heart attacks and strokes. Think of it like repeatedly revving a car engine in neutral—eventually, this constant strain damages the heart and blood vessels. The heart isn't designed to handle these frequent stress responses during what should be a time of rest and recovery. This explains why untreated sleep apnea patients often develop irregular heart rhythms and have a significantly higher risk of heart failure. Even mild sleep apnea can increase cardiovascular risk, and the risk grows substantially as the condition becomes more severe.

The effects on brain function can be equally serious [18]. Recent research shows that untreated sleep apnea may accelerate cognitive decline, potentially hastening the onset of conditions like mild cognitive impairment and Alzheimer's disease by up to a decade. For older adults, this means sleep apnea might not just make them tired—it could actually speed up brain aging. The connection appears to work through several mechanisms. First, the repeated oxygen drops may directly damage brain cells [19]. Second, the fragmented sleep prevents the brain from performing its crucial nighttime maintenance, including clearing out toxic proteins that can accumulate and contribute to neurodegeneration. Third, the constant stress responses and inflammation can damage small blood vessels in the brain. Even in younger people, untreated sleep apnea can impair memory, attention, and decision-making abilities, affecting everything from job performance to personal relationships.

Sleep apnea's influence on metabolism helps explain its connection to type 2 diabetes [18]. The repeated drops in oxygen and disrupted sleep patterns interfere with how the body processes sugar, leading to insulin resistance. It's like having a faulty thermostat—even though insulin is available, the body can't use it effectively to regulate blood sugar levels. This metabolic disruption can either increase diabetes risk or make existing diabetes harder to control. The relationship works both ways—poor sleep affects hormones that control appetite and metabolism, leading to weight gain, which in turn can worsen sleep apnea. Additionally, the stress responses triggered by sleep apnea cause the body to release stress hormones like cortisol, which further disrupts blood sugar control and can contribute to increased belly fat—a shared risk factor for both sleep apnea and diabetes.

Perhaps most surprising is the emerging evidence linking untreated sleep apnea to increased cancer risk, particularly for certain types like colorectal and breast cancers, through the increase in risk is not large [20]. Scientists believe the repeated oxygen deprivation and resulting inflammation might create conditions that promote tumor growth. While this connection requires further research, it adds urgency to the importance of treating sleep apnea promptly.

Mental health also suffers when sleep apnea goes untreated [21]. The constant sleep disruption affects the brain's ability to regulate mood, potentially triggering or worsening depression and anxiety. Untreated sleep apnea can trap people in a cycle—poor sleep worsens mood, which in turn makes it harder to cope with stress or seek help.

The good news is that treating sleep apnea can reverse or prevent many of these complications. CPAP therapy, for instance, not only improves sleep quality but also helps reduce blood pressure, enhance mood, and improve cognitive function [22, 23]. Even in cases where some damage has occurred, proper treatment can help reduce the risk of further progression. Understanding these long-term consequences emphasizes why treating sleep apnea promptly matters so much. While the immediate symptoms of daytime sleepiness and loud snoring might seem merely inconvenient, the potential long-term impact on health makes early diagnosis and treatment more important than ever.

References

1. Gottlieb DJ, Punjabi NM. Diagnosis and management of obstructive sleep apnea: a review. JAMA. 2020;323(14):1389–400. PMID: 32286648.
2. Won CHJ, Qin L, Selim B, Yaggi HK. Varying hypopnea definitions affect obstructive sleep apnea severity classification and association with cardiovascular disease. J Clin Sleep Med. 2018;14(12):1987–94. PMID: 30518445.
3. Abbasi A, Gupta SS, Sabharwal N, Meghrajani V, Sharma S, Kamholz S, Kupfer Y. A comprehensive review of obstructive sleep apnea. Sleep Sci. 2021;14(2):142–54. PMID: 34381578.
4. Fattal D, Hester S, Wendt L. Body weight and obstructive sleep apnea: a mathematical relationship between body mass index and apnea-hypopnea index in veterans. J Clin Sleep Med. 2022;18(12):2723–9. PMID: 35929587.
5. Haradwala MB, Sivaraman M. Largest neck circumference associated with obstructive sleep apnea: a case report. Cureus. 2024;16(2):e54761. PMID: 38524094.
6. Ghimire P, Sankari A, Antoine MH, et al. Obesity-hypoventilation syndrome. Updated 2024 Feb 3. In: StatPearls [Internet]. Treasure Island: StatPearls; 2025 Jan. https://www.ncbi.nlm.nih.gov/books/NBK542216/
7. Badr MS, Dingell JD, Javaheri S. Central sleep apnea: a brief review. Curr Pulmonol Rep. 2019;8(1):14–21. PMID: 31788413.
8. Terziyski K, Draganova A. Central sleep apnea with cheyne-stokes breathing in heart failure – from research to clinical practice and beyond. Adv Exp Med Biol. 2018;1067:327–51. PMID: 29411336.
9. Rudrappa M, Modi P, Bollu PC. Cheyne stokes respirations. [Updated 2023 Jul 31]. In: StatPearls [Internet]. Treasure Island: StatPearls; 2025 Jan. https://www.ncbi.nlm.nih.gov/books/NBK448165/
10. Khan MT, Franco RA. Complex sleep apnea syndrome. 2014;2014:798487. PMID: 24693440.
11. Romero-Corral A, Caples SM, Lopez-Jimenez F, Somers VK. Interactions between obesity and obstructive sleep apnea: implications for treatment. Chest. 2010;137(3):711–9. PMID: 20202954.
12. Janney CA, Kilbourne AM, Germain A, Lai Z, Hoerster KD, Goodrich DE, Klingaman EA, Verchinina L, Richardson CR. The influence of sleep disordered breathing on weight loss in a national weight management program. Sleep. 2016;39(1):59–65. PMID: 26350475.
13. Li M, Lin H, Yang Q, Zhang X, Zhou Q, Shi J, Ge F. Glucagon-like peptide 1 receptor agonists for the treatment of obstructive sleep apnea:a meta-analysis. Sleep. 2024;29:zsae280. PMID: 39626095.
14. Puhan MA, Suarez A, Lo Cascio C, Zahn A, Heitz M, Braendli O. Didgeridoo playing as alternative treatment for obstructive sleep apnoea syndrome: randomised controlled trial. BMJ. 2006;332(7536):266–70. PMID: 16377643.
15. Mashaqi S, Patel SI, Combs D, Estep L, Helmick S, Machamer J, Parthasarathy S. The hypoglossal nerve stimulation as a novel therapy for treating obstructive sleep apnea-a literature review. Int J Environ Res Public Health. 2021;18(4):1642. PMID: 33572156.
16. Sheen D, Abdulateef S. Uvulopalatopharyngoplasty. Oral Maxillofac Surg Clin North Am. 2021;33(2):295–303. PMID: 33581977.
17. Cerritelli L, Caranti A, Migliorelli A, Bianchi G, Stringa LM, Bonsembiante A, Cammaroto G, Pelucchi S, Vicini C. Sleep position and obstructive sleep apnea (OSA): do we know how we sleep? A new explorative sleeping questionnaire. Sleep Breath. 2022;26(4):1973–81. PMID: 35129756.
18. Knauert M, Naik S, Gillespie MB, Kryger M. Clinical consequences and economic costs of untreated obstructive sleep apnea syndrome. World J Otorhinolaryngol Head Neck Surg. 2015;1(1):17–27. PMID: 29204536.
19. UCLA Health. Want to protect your brain? Treat your obstructive sleep apnea [Internet]. Los Angeles: University of California Los Angeles Health; Cited 2024 Jan 26. https://www.uclahealth.org/news/article/want-protect-your-brain-treat-your-obstructive-sleep-apnea

20. Cheng L, Guo H, Zhang Z, Yao Y, Yao Q. Obstructive sleep apnea and incidence of malignant tumors: a meta-analysis. Sleep Med. 2021;84:195-04. https://doi.org/10.1016/j.sleep.2021.05.029
21. Gupta MA, Simpson FC. Obstructive sleep apnea and psychiatric disorders: a systematic review. J Clin Sleep Med. 2015;11(2):165–75. PMID: 25406268.
22. Wickwire EM, Bailey MD, Somers VK, Srivastava MC, Scharf SM, Johnson AM, Albrecht JS. CPAP adherence reduces cardiovascular risk among older adults with obstructive sleep apnea. Sleep Breath. 2021;25(3):1343–50. PMID: 33141315.
23. Seda G, Matwiyoff G, Parrish JS. Effects of obstructive sleep apnea and CPAP on cognitive function. Curr Neurol Neurosci Rep. 2021;21(7):32. PMID: 33956247.

Restless Leg Syndrome and Periodic Limb Movement Disorder

23

23.1 When Legs Won't Rest: Restless Legs Syndrome and Periodic Limb Movement Disorder

23.1.1 What Are Restless Legs Syndrome and Periodic Limb Movement Disorder?

Among sleep disorders, Restless Legs Syndrome (RLS) stands out for its distinctive and often maddening symptoms. Imagine feeling an irresistible urge to move your legs just as you're trying to relax in bed—sensations that are describe as crawling, tingling, itching, or even electric-like discomfort that are usually only relieved by movement. This condition, producing clinically significant symptoms in at least 2–3% of adults and up to 1% of children, typically strikes in the evening or at night when you're just about to fall asleep, transforming the simple act of falling asleep into a significant challenge [1].

The experience of RLS is both distinctive and frustrating. Just as someone tries to settle down for the evening—perhaps while watching television or lying in bed—these uncomfortable sensations begin creeping through their legs [1]. Walking, stretching, or moving the legs provides relief, but the discomfort in some cases returns as soon as they rest again. It's as if the legs have a mind of their own, demanding movement when the rest of the body craves stillness. This pattern helps explain why doctors use the acronym "URGE" to capture RLS's main features: the Urge to move, Rest-induced symptoms, Getting better with activity, and Evening worsening.

While the causes of RLS and Periodic Limb Movement Disorder (PLMD) are not fully understood, reduced levels of dopamine, a crucial brain chemical that helps control movement, play an important role. When dopamine systems don't function properly, the brain can't regulate movement normally, leading to the uncomfortable sensations and urges that characterize RLS. This may explain both why movement temporarily helps—it briefly increases dopamine activity—and why the relief in some cases is so short-lived, creating that frustrating pattern of

A. Juginović, *Sleep Science Made Simple*,
https://doi.org/10.1007/978-3-031-92060-8_23

needing to move again and again. Iron plays a surprisingly important role in this system too [1]. It serves as an essential building block for producing dopamine in the brain. When iron levels fall too low, it disrupts dopamine function, potentially triggering or worsening RLS symptoms. This connection helps explain several aspects of RLS—why iron supplements help many patients, why pregnant women (who often develop iron deficiency) frequently experience RLS during their third trimester, and why blood tests for iron levels are often one of the first steps in diagnosis. It also helps explain why some Parkinson's disease patients experience RLS, as both conditions involve dopamine system disruption. Genetics add another layer to the story—about 40% (and even up to 90%) of RLS cases run in families [2, 3]. While pregnancy-related RLS typically resolves after delivery when iron levels normalize, people with genetic predisposition often experience symptoms throughout their lives, though severity can vary significantly over time.

RLS appears in two distinct patterns that help guide treatment. Early-onset RLS, beginning before age 45, often runs in families and may gradually worsen over time [2]. These patients typically need more aggressive treatment approaches. Late-onset RLS, appearing after 45, typically arrives more suddenly but doesn't usually progress as dramatically [2]. Often, treating underlying conditions like iron deficiency can significantly improve symptoms in these cases.

While RLS occurs when you're awake, many patients also experience a related condition during sleep called Periodic Limb Movement Disorder (PLMD) [1]. Unlike RLS, which involves conscious urges to move, PLMD causes involuntary leg or arm movements—usually brief twitches or jerks—every 20–40 seconds during sleep. These movements often go unnoticed by the person but are frequently observed by a bed partner as repetitive kicking or jerking.

PLMD is best detected during sleep studies, where electrodes placed on leg muscles detect these leg movements. The movements typically occur in clusters during lighter sleep stages and can happen hundreds of times per night. Interestingly, during REM sleep, when the brain naturally paralyzes most muscles to prevent dream enactment, these movements typically cease. About 80% of people with RLS also have PLMD, but not everyone with PLMD has RLS. This overlap suggests the two may share similar disruptions in the brain's motor control systems [4].

These repetitive movements can fragment sleep—even if the person doesn't fully wake up. Each movement can cause a brief arousal, interrupting deeper sleep stages. This explains why people with PLMD often feel unrested despite seemingly sleeping through the night. The repeated arousals can lead to daytime fatigue, difficulty concentrating, and mood changes—similar to the effects of other sleep disorders that fragment sleep.

23.1.2 Treatment Options

Treating these conditions often begins with investigating underlying causes and making lifestyle modifications [1]. Blood tests can reveal iron deficiency (through measuring serum ferritin, a protein that stores iron in the body), which is a common and treatable trigger for RLS and PLMD. Regular exercise (though not too close to bedtime), reducing caffeine and alcohol intake, and maintaining consistent sleep schedules can help manage mild symptoms. Some people find relief through specific activities during episodes—walking, stretching, hot baths, or leg massages.

When these approaches are insufficient, several medication options exist [1]. The most common medications (like ropinirole or pramipexole) work by adjusting levels of dopamine—the brain chemical that helps control movement. However, some patients find these medications become less effective over time or even make symptoms worse, a problem doctors call "augmentation". Other options include medications typically used for nerve pain (like gabapentin) that can be particularly helpful for people who experience painful sensations. In severe cases where other treatments don't work, doctors might prescribe a benzodiazepine like clonazepam or pain medications. For PLMD, doctors can prescribe muscle relaxants (like baclofen) or anti-seizure medications (like gabapentin or pregabalin) to reduce the leg movements during sleep. Finding the right treatment often requires patience and careful monitoring.

Living with RLS or PLMD affects more than just nighttime comfort—these conditions can interfere with daily routines, relationships, and overall quality of life. People with RLS often structure their days around their symptoms—avoiding long car trips, choosing aisle seats at movies, or declining evening social events because they know they'll need to keep moving. Some find themselves pacing their bedroom for hours, fighting the uncomfortable sensations that prevent sleep. The sleep disruption can create particular challenges for couples. A partner's repeated leg movements during sleep might force couples to sleep separately, affecting their relationship intimacy. Sometimes, the person with PLMD remains unaware of their nighttime movements until their partner describes the constant kicking or jerking that disrupts both people's sleep.

While these conditions might not receive as much attention as sleep apnea or insomnia, their impact on quality of life can be equally significant. The good news is that with proper diagnosis and treatment, most people can find significant relief from their symptoms, allowing them to return to restful sleep and more comfortable days.

References

1. Kouri I, Junna MR, Lipford MC. Restless legs syndrome and periodic limb movements of sleep: from neurophysiology to clinical practice. J Clin Neurophysiol. 2023;40(3):215–23. PMID: 36872500.
2. Didato G, Di Giacomo R, Rosa GJ, Dominese A, de Curtis M, Lanteri P. Restless legs syndrome across the lifespan: symptoms, pathophysiology, management and daily life impact of the different patterns of disease presentation. Int J Environ Res Public Health. 2020;17(10):3658. PMID: 32456058.
3. Winkelmann J, Ferini-Strambi L. Genetics of restless legs syndrome. Sleep Med Rev. 2006;10(3):179–83. PMID: 16624598.
4. Doan TT, Koo BB, Ogilvie RP, Redline S, Lutsey PL. Restless legs syndrome and periodic limb movements during sleep in the multi-ethnic study of atherosclerosis. Sleep. 2018;41(8):zsy106. PMID: 29860522.

Circadian Rhythm Disorders 24

24.1 Circadian Rhythm Disorders: When Your Body's Clock Is Disrupted

24.1.1 Introduction

Have you ever noticed how jet lag can leave you alert at 3 AM or nodding off during an afternoon meeting? For most people, these temporary disruptions resolve within a few days. But for those with circadian rhythm disorders, this misalignment between their body's internal clock and the external world becomes a constant struggle. These disorders occur when your body's master clock—the brain's suprachiasmatic nucleus (SCN) we discussed earlier in the book—fails to properly synchronize with the 24-h day. While occasional poor sleep is common, people with circadian disorders experience ongoing shifts in their entire sleep-wake cycle, making it biologically difficult to maintain typical sleep and wake times.

Several factors can contribute to circadian rhythm disorders [1]. Genetics plays a significant role—specific mutations in "clock genes" can cause our internal timing to run faster or slower than 24 h [2]. These inherited differences explain why circadian disorders often run in families and why they typically appear during adolescence or early adulthood. Brain injury or disease can also disrupt circadian timing by affecting the neural pathways that connect your eyes to the SCN, preventing proper processing of light signals—the main time cue that keeps our internal clock synchronized. Finally, psychiatric illnesses or external stressors can also influence our ability to maintain an optimal 24-h rhythm.

Age affects our circadian system too. During adolescence, biological changes naturally delay sleep timing—explaining why teenagers typically become "night owls." As we age, this pattern often reverses, leading to earlier sleep and wake times. Environmental factors can also trigger or worsen these disorders, particularly irregular exposure to light and darkness or social demands that force us to ignore our body's natural timing.

A. Juginović, *Sleep Science Made Simple*,
https://doi.org/10.1007/978-3-031-92060-8_24

Circadian rhythm disorders can be grouped into several distinct patterns, each with unique effects on sleep timing:

- Delayed Sleep Phase Disorder (DSPD), the most common type, creates a persistent pattern of late sleeping and waking [1]. People with DSPD (more common in younger people) might find their natural sleep time falls between 3 AM and 11 AM, even when they need to be awake earlier. Despite feeling exhausted during the day, they find it biologically impossible to fall asleep at conventional bedtimes—their sleep drive simply doesn't activate until much later.
- Advanced Sleep Phase Disorder (ASPD) presents the opposite pattern—overwhelming sleepiness in early evening and very early morning awakening [1]. Someone with ASPD might naturally fall asleep at 7 PM and wake at 3 AM. While this pattern might accommodate early work schedules, it can severely limit evening activities and social life.
- Non-24-Hour Sleep-Wake Disorder involves a constantly shifting sleep pattern [1]. Unlike DSPD or ASPD, which maintain a consistent (though shifted) schedule, here the circadian pacemaker is unable to synchronize with the 24-h day. This results in a progressive delay or advance of sleep-wake times, leading to periodic nighttime insomnia and daytime sleepiness as the individual's sleep-wake cycle drifts in and out of alignment with the 24-h day. This condition primarily affects blind individuals who in most cases cannot receive the light signals necessary for circadian entrainment.
- Irregular Sleep-Wake Rhythm Disorder represents the most severe disruption of circadian timing [1]. Instead of any consistent pattern, sleep fragments into multiple short episodes throughout the day and night. This condition typically occurs in people with neurodegenerative diseases or severe brain injuries, highlighting how crucial intact neural circuits are for maintaining regular sleep-wake patterns.

24.1.2 Diagnostic and Treatment Approaches: Resetting the Biological Clock

Diagnosing circadian rhythm disorders requires detailed evaluation to distinguish them from other sleep-related conditions, especially those involving insomnia or irregular sleep habits [1]. Sleep specialists typically start with a detailed sleep history, often asking patients to maintain a sleep diary for several weeks. These diaries track not just sleep times but also daily activities, light exposure, and meals, revealing patterns that patients might not notice themselves. For some patients, actigraphy—using a wrist-worn device that tracks activity levels—helps document sleep-wake cycles over extended periods. While traditional overnight sleep studies aren't usually necessary, they might be used to rule out other sleep disorders.

The timing of sleep isn't the only consideration—doctors also evaluate how the sleep pattern affects daily functioning and whether the pattern causes distress. Blood tests might check for underlying conditions affecting sleep timing, like thyroid problems. Understanding family history proves particularly important since many circadian disorders run in families.

Treatment for circadian disorders focuses on realigning the internal clock with the external world through a combination of carefully timed interventions. Unlike general sleep problems where simple sleep hygiene changes might suffice, circadian disorders require precise timing of both light exposure and medications to effectively shift sleep patterns.

Light therapy is often the first line treatment, but timing is crucial [1]. Light works by directly signaling to your SCN through specialized cells in your retina, which then influences both the immediate suppression of melatonin and the timing of future melatonin release. For Delayed Sleep Phase Disorder, bright light exposure in the early morning helps reset the delayed clock by suppressing any remaining melatonin left over during the night and shifting the next day's melatonin release earlier. However, someone with Advanced Sleep Phase Disorder needs evening light exposure to delay their melatonin release to a later time. The wrong timing can actually worsen the misalignment—just as using bright screens in the evening can disrupt normal sleep patterns by confusing these light-sensitive pathways.

Melatonin supplementation also requires precise timing [1]. Unlike its general use for sleep problems, treating circadian disorders means taking melatonin at specific times based on your type of disorder. Someone with Delayed Sleep Phase Disorder might need melatonin several hours before their desired bedtime to help advance their sleep phase. For Advanced Sleep Phase Disorder, melatonin timing shifts to the early morning to help delay sleep onset the following evening.

People with Non-24-Hour Sleep-Wake Disorder or Irregular Sleep-Wake Rhythm Disorder often need more intensive management approaches apart from melatonin and bright light, sometimes including scheduled activities throughout the day to help strengthen circadian signals. These cases frequently require collaboration between sleep specialists and other healthcare providers, particularly when underlying conditions contribute to the disorder.

Strict consistency in sleep schedules is crucial to reinforcing these biological interventions. Even minor deviations can undo weeks of careful timing adjustments. This means:

- Keeping the same sleep and wake times every day, even on weekends.
- Creating a completely dark sleep environment.
- Carefully timing exercise and meals to support desired sleep patterns.
- Avoiding bright light exposure during times when it could worsen circadian misalignment.

The social and professional impact of these disorders often requires lifestyle adaptations. Some people find success by adjusting work schedules to better match their biological rhythms—for instance, someone with Delayed Sleep Phase Disorder might perform better with a later work schedule. Managing these disorders becomes particularly challenging for blind individuals with Non-24-Hour Sleep-Wake Disorder or people with neurodegenerative conditions who have Irregular Sleep-Wake Rhythm Disorder. These cases often require more intensive approaches and coordination between sleep specialists and other healthcare providers.

Recent advances in chronotherapy—the timing of treatments based on the body's circadian rhythms—have improved treatment outcomes. However, success requires understanding that these represent real medical conditions requiring systematic treatment approaches, not just poor sleep habits. With proper diagnosis and consistent treatment, most people can achieve better alignment between their internal clock and external demands, though some may need to adapt their lifestyle to work with, rather than against, their biological timing.

References

1. Steele TA, St Louis EK, Videnovic A, Auger RR. Circadian rhythm sleep-wake disorders: a contemporary review of neurobiology, treatment, and dysregulation in neurodegenerative disease. Neurotherapeutics. 2021;18(1):53–74. PMID: 33844152.
2. Rijo-Ferreira F, Takahashi JS. Genomics of circadian rhythms in health and disease. Genome Med. 2019;11(1):82. PMID: 31847894.

Parasomnias 25

25.1 Parasomnias: When Sleep Gets Strange

25.1.1 Introduction to Parasomnias

Throughout this book, we've discussed disorders that affect falling asleep or staying asleep. Parasomnias pose a different kind of sleep challenge—these disorders involve unusual behaviors and experiences that occur during sleep itself, often without any conscious awareness [1]. During parasomnia episodes, some brain regions remain in sleep mode while others become partially activated, leading to complex behaviors. Think of parasomnias as disorders of "mixed states," where boundaries between sleep and wakefulness blur. In non-REM parasomnias, the body can move and act while the brain remains in deep sleep, allowing complex behaviors like walking or eating [1]. REM parasomnias, on the other hand, occur when the normal muscle paralysis during REM sleep fails, letting people physically act out their dreams, sometimes with dramatic or dangerous consequences [1].

The prevalence of different parasomnias varies significantly—while up to 6.5% of children experience sleep terrors, REM Sleep Behavior Disorder (RBD) affects less than 1% of adults [2, 3]. However, all these disorders share a common theme: they reveal how complex sleep really is, and how different parts of our brain can operate semi-independently during sleep.

The timing of parasomnias directly relates to our sleep architecture—the pattern of sleep stages we discussed earlier. Non-REM parasomnias typically occur during deep sleep in the first third of the night, when stage N3 (deep sleep) predominates. During this period, your brain oscillates between lighter and deeper sleep states, creating brief moments when some brain regions can become partially awakened while others remain in deep sleep. This explains why these events often occur 1–3 h after falling asleep, when deep sleep reaches its peak.

REM-related parasomnias, in contrast, emerge during REM or "dream sleep" in the latter part of the night, when REM periods become longer and more frequent. Remember how REM sleep normally paralyzes our muscles to prevent dream

A. Juginović, *Sleep Science Made Simple*,
https://doi.org/10.1007/978-3-031-92060-8_25

enactment? REM parasomnias occur when this protective mechanism fails, allowing physical movements during dream sleep. This timing explains why episodes tend to occur in the early morning hours, when REM sleep is much more frequent.

25.1.2 Non-REM Parasomnias

Sleepwalking (somnambulism) occurs during deep sleep and can involve surprisingly complex activities [1]. Sleepwalkers might walk around their home, rearrange objects, eat, or in rare cases even drive—all while their brain remains primarily in deep sleep. While waking a sleepwalker won't cause harm (contrary to popular belief), the real danger comes from potential injuries during their unconscious activities. Up to 15% of children experience sleepwalking, though most outgrow it by adolescence [4].

Sleep terrors demonstrate how powerfully emotions can emerge during sleep [2]. Unlike nightmares that occur during REM sleep, sleep terrors erupt from deep sleep with sudden screaming, intense fear, and racing heartbeat. People having sleep terrors might bolt upright in bed, appear terrified, and be inconsolable for several minutes. Despite how dramatic these episodes appear, people typically have no memory of them the next morning. Like sleepwalking, sleep terrors are more common in children.

25.1.3 REM Parasomnias

REM Sleep Behavior Disorder (RBD) occurs when normal muscle paralysis during this stage of sleep fails [5]. People with RBD physically act out their dreams—they might punch, kick, or leap out of bed while dreaming about fighting or running. These behaviors can cause injury to both the person and their bed partner. RBD deserves particular attention because it often appears years before certain neurodegenerative conditions, especially Parkinson's disease, making it an important early warning sign. Unlike most parasomnias, RBD typically affects older adults and is more common in men.

25.1.4 Other Sleep-Related Behaviors

Several other parasomnias can occur across different stages of sleep [1]. Sleep talking ranges from simple mumbling to complex conversations, though speakers rarely remember these episodes. Sleep-related eating disorder involves consuming food while in a semi-conscious or unconscious state, sometimes even including inedible or dangerous items. Teeth grinding, or bruxism, often goes unnoticed until dental damage becomes apparent or bed partners complain about the noise. Sleep-related groaning, called catathrenia, produces loud moaning sounds during sleep that can be disturbing to bed partners.

Sleep paralysis occurs when the muscle atonia of REM sleep temporarily persists into wakefulness, creating a frightening experience of being unable to move while fully conscious [6]. During these episodes, which typically last seconds to a few minutes, people remain fully aware of their surroundings but cannot move or speak. Many experience a sensation of pressure on their chest and difficulty breathing. Some people also report frightening hallucinations—seeing or sensing a presence in the room, hearing sounds, or feeling touched. These hallucinations likely represent dream activity continuing into wakefulness, similar to how muscle paralysis persists. Sleep paralysis occurs more frequently when sleep patterns are irregular or during sleep deprivation, and episodes often run in families. Although often frightening, sleep paralysis is generally harmless and resolves on its own as the brain completes its transition to wakefulness.

25.1.5 Diagnosing and Treating Parasomnias

Diagnosing parasomnias begins with a careful clinical history, often involving input from both patients and their bed partners in order to document when episodes occur and what behaviors they involve [1]. Video recordings from home can provide valuable information about the timing and nature of events. In some cases, overnight sleep studies (polysomnography) may be needed. During these studies, sleep specialists usually monitor brain waves, muscle activity, breathing patterns, and video recordings to capture parasomnia episodes and determine during which sleep stage they occur. This helps distinguish between different types of parasomnias and rule out other sleep disorders (or other medical conditions) that might cause similar behaviors.

Treatment approaches vary depending on the specific parasomnia and its underlying causes [1]. For sleepwalking and sleep terrors, safety becomes the primary concern. This means securing the sleep environment—installing locks on windows and doors, removing hazardous objects, and sometimes using alarms or motion sensors. REM Sleep Behavior Disorder often responds well to medications like clonazepam and melatonin, which help suppress motor activity during REM sleep and reduce the frequency of dream enactment behaviors. For teeth grinding, dental appliances can protect against damage while medications and stress reduction techniques might help reduce the behavior.

Many parasomnias, particularly in children, resolve naturally with time [1]. For adults, treating underlying conditions or factors often proves crucial. This includes managing stress, maintaining regular sleep schedules, avoiding sleep deprivation, and addressing any other sleep disorders that might trigger parasomnia episodes. Certain medications can trigger or worsen parasomnias, so reviewing and adjusting medications sometimes helps reduce episodes.

Some people benefit from specific behavioral therapies. For sleepwalking, scheduled awakenings—waking someone shortly before their typical episode time—can help break the pattern. Relaxation techniques and stress management often reduce episode frequency for various parasomnias. People with REM Sleep Behavior Disorder might need to adapt their sleep environment, perhaps using padded bed rails or sleeping in separate beds to prevent injury.

While parasomnias can seem dramatic or frightening, proper diagnosis and treatment allow most people to manage their condition effectively. The key lies in understanding that these represent treatable medical conditions, not psychological problems or character flaws. With appropriate intervention, both the affected person and their bed partner can return to peaceful, safe sleep.

References

1. Singh S, Kaur H, Singh S, Khawaja I. Parasomnias: a comprehensive review. Cureus. 2018;10(12):e3807. PMID: 30868021.
2. Leung AKC, Leung AAM, Wong AHC, Hon KL. Sleep terrors: an updated review. Curr Pediatr Rev. 2020;16(3):176–182. PMID: 31612833.
3. Khawaja I, Spurling BC, Singh S. REM sleep behavior disorder. [Updated 2023 Apr 24]. In: StatPearls [Internet]. Treasure Island: StatPearls; 2025 Jan. https://www.ncbi.nlm.nih.gov/books/NBK534239/
4. Fariba KA, Tadi P. Parasomnias. [Updated 2023 Jul 17]. In: StatPearls [Internet]. Treasure Island: StatPearls; 2025 Jan. https://www.ncbi.nlm.nih.gov/books/NBK560524/
5. Khawaja I, Spurling BC, Singh S. REM sleep behavior disorder. 2023 Apr 24. In: StatPearls [Internet]. Treasure Island: StatPearls; 2025 Jan. PMID: 30480972.
6. Farooq M, Anjum F. Sleep paralysis. 2023 Sep 4. In: StatPearls [Internet]. Treasure Island: StatPearls; 2025 Jan. PMID: 32965993.

Better Sleep at Home 26

26.1 Optimizing Your Sleep at Home

Throughout this book, we've explored the science of sleep—from the neural circuits regulating your sleep-wake cycles to the mechanisms underlying various sleep disorders. We've seen how your brain's master clock orchestrates daily rhythms and how different sleep stages serve vital biological functions. In this section, we'll briefly recap some of the key concepts, while pointing you to earlier chapters for a deeper dive into the details. Now it's time to translate this scientific understanding into practical strategies for better sleep.

Environmental Factors

Temperature plays a critical role in sleep quality. Your bedroom temperature directly affects your body's natural thermoregulation during sleep. The ideal sleeping temperature falls between 15 and 20 °C (60–67 °F). Warmer temperatures can hinder your body's natural nighttime cooling process, making both sleep onset and maintenance more difficult.

Light exposure directly influences sleep timing by acting on the suprachiasmatic nucleus (SCN). Evening light and light during sleep, especially from electronic devices, suppresses melatonin production and activates wake-promoting circuits. Even brief exposure to blue light can disrupt your sleep timing system. Reducing light exposure, particularly from screens, at least an hour before bedtime, as well as keeping the room dark during sleep helps maintain proper melatonin production. Finally, exposing yourself to natural morning light can help reset your circadian rhythm.

Timing and Consistency

Keeping consistent sleep and wake times helps reinforce your circadian rhythms, the internal biological cycles that regulate sleep and many other body functions. Even small shifts in your schedule—like sleeping in on weekends—can disrupt these rhythms, a phenomenon known as social jet lag, a mismatch between your

A. Juginović, *Sleep Science Made Simple*,
https://doi.org/10.1007/978-3-031-92060-8_26

body's internal clock and your social schedule, similar to the effects of travel jet lag. This misalignment between your internal clock and daily obligations can negatively affect sleep quality, mood, and overall health.

Daily Habits and Sleep

Certain substances can profoundly impact sleep quality by altering brain activity. Caffeine, found in coffee, tea, and energy drinks, blocks adenosine from binding to its receptors. This is crucial as adenosine is natural chemical that makes us feel sleepy as it builds up in the brain throughout the day. By interfering with this process, caffeine delays sleep onset and makes sleep lighter, with its stimulating effects lasting 4–8 h. Although alcohol may help you fall asleep initially, it disrupts sleep in the second half of the night. It breaks up sleep cycles and particularly suppresses REM sleep, the stage important for processing emotions and storing memories, often leaving sleep fragmented and unrefreshing.

Nutrition and Sleep

The timing of your meal can significantly influence sleep quality. Large meals eaten within 2–3 h of bedtime raise core body temperature and stimulate digestion at a time when your body should be cooling down in preparation for sleep. Small evening snacks combining tryptophan-rich foods (turkey, eggs, dairy) with complex carbohydrates may support sleep by promoting serotonin and melatonin production. Some foods, including kiwis, tart cherries, and fatty fish, may improve sleep quality through their nutrient profiles. While supplements like melatonin, magnesium, L-theanine, and valerian root show some evidence of effectiveness, their effects vary between individuals.

Exercise and Light Exposure

Regular exercise promotes better sleep through multiple mechanisms, but timing matters. Since vigorous exercise raises core body temperature and stress hormone levels, it is not recommended very close to bedtime. Morning workouts, especially outdoors, offer the added benefit of natural light exposure, which helps synchronize your circadian rhythms. Seasonal changes require adjusting exercise timing—morning outdoor exercise becomes particularly valuable during winter months when natural light exposure decreases (Fig. 26.1).

Strategic Napping

Short naps can help boost alertness and fight daytime sleepiness without harming nighttime sleep—if timed correctly. The ideal nap lasts 20–30 min (between 2 PM and 4 PM), long enough to recharge energy without entering deeper sleep stages that cause grogginess and can ruin you nighttime sleep. Napping before 3–4 PM prevents it from interfering with the natural sleep pressure that builds throughout the day. An effective trick is the "coffee nap"(sometimes called a "nappuccino"): drinking coffee just before a short nap allows you to wake up as the caffeine kicks in, combining the benefits of both for maximum alertness. However, longer naps—over 30 min—are more likely to cause sleep inertia (that sluggish feeling after waking) and can reduce your need for sleep at night, making it harder to fall asleep later.

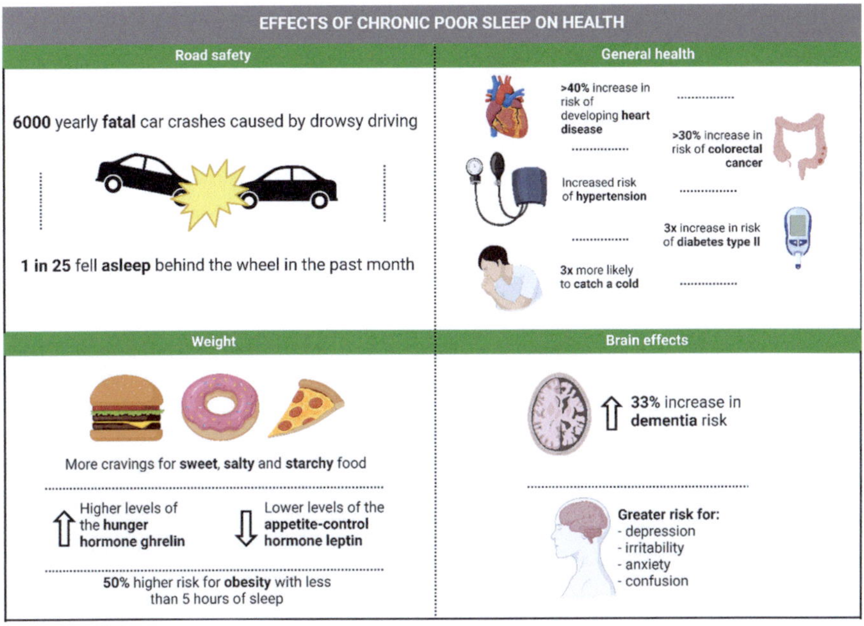

Fig. 26.1 Wide-ranging health impacts of poor sleep. ("Created in BioRender. Juginovic, A. (2025) https://BioRender.com/x14v509")

Practical Sleep Strategies

Several evidence-based approaches can help when sleep proves difficult. Maintaining a consistent pre-sleep routine helps condition your brain for sleep. If sleep doesn't come within 20 min, temporarily leaving the bed prevents developing negative associations with your sleep environment. Avoid checking the time during night awakenings, as this often triggers anxiety and activates arousal systems. Your physical sleep environment significantly affects sleep quality. Your mattress and pillows need to support proper body alignment for optimal muscle relaxation and parasympathetic system activation. Using your bed only for sleep and intimacy strengthens the association between your sleep environment and sleep itself.

Specific relaxation techniques can help your body shift from the "fight or flight" state of stress to the "rest and digest" mode needed for sleep. One simple method is progressive muscle relaxation, which helps release physical tension and quiet the mind. Right before going to sleep, you can start by tensing the muscles in your feet for a few seconds, then slowly relax them, noticing the difference between tension and relaxation. Then, move upward through your body—legs, stomach, chest, arms—until you reach your head, letting each muscle group soften. This practice not only relieves built-up tension but also helps anchor your attention to your body rather than racing thoughts. Another effective technique is the 4–7-8 breathing method. Inhale gently through your nose for 4 s, hold your breath for 7 s, and exhale slowly through your mouth for 8 s. Repeating this cycle for a few minutes slows your heart rate, signals your body to relax, and creates a natural sense of calm.

Practicing either of these methods for 5–10 min before bed can make it easier to fall asleep, especially if your mind feels busy at night.

When sleep difficulties persist despite implementing these measures, consult a healthcare provider. Sleep disorders represent real medical conditions requiring proper evaluation and treatment, as their effects extend throughout the body's biological systems. Understanding and applying sleep science principles allows most people to achieve better sleep quality, but knowing when to seek professional help proves equally important for optimal sleep health.

Future of Sleep Science 27

27.1 Looking Forward: The Future of Sleep Science and Medicine

Sleep science continues to develop with new technologies revealing additional aspects of brain activity during sleep, while genetic research helps clarify how our DNA influences sleep patterns. These advances help explain individual differences in sleep disorders and highlight why treatment approaches often require personalization. Artificial intelligence (AI) and machine learning applications represent significant developments in sleep research and clinical practice. These AI systems can analyze large datasets from sleep studies to identify subtle patterns that human observers might miss. For example, certain EEG signatures might predict who will develop specific sleep disorders, or which patients will respond best to particular treatments. As AI algorithms improve, they may help provide more accurate sleep staging and disorder classification than traditional manual scoring methods.

The relationship between sleep and aging is receiving increased attention as populations grow older in many countries. Researchers are studying how sleep quality might relate to cognitive health with age, particularly how the brain's waste clearance processes during sleep may affect protein accumulation associated with certain neurological conditions. This work raises questions about whether maintaining good sleep habits throughout life might contribute to brain health in later years.

Environmental factors present considerations for sleep researchers to address. Temperature changes related to climate patterns can affect the body temperature decreases normally associated with sleep onset, while increasing artificial light exposure can influence natural sleep timing for many organisms, including humans. For people, exposure to light, particularly blue wavelengths from screens and newer lighting, can affect melatonin production and potentially disrupt normal sleep timing. Understanding these environmental factors becomes more important as we consider their potential effects on sleep patterns.

A. Juginović, *Sleep Science Made Simple*,
https://doi.org/10.1007/978-3-031-92060-8_27

Work patterns continue to change, with remote and flexible schedules becoming more common. These changes create opportunities to potentially align work times with individual sleep preferences, but also present challenges as technology can blur boundaries between work and personal time. Researchers are studying how these evolving work arrangements might affect sleep-wake cycles and how schedules might be optimized to support both productivity and adequate rest.

Treatment approaches for sleep disorders continue to develop beyond traditional methods. New technologies like virtual reality systems might help create environments conducive to sleep onset, while improvements in light therapy could provide more options for addressing circadian rhythm disruptions. Artificial intelligence is beginning to influence treatment approaches as well. AI systems can analyze patterns in an individual's sleep and activity data to recommend optimal sleep schedules and behavioral interventions tailored to their specific needs. Some emerging applications use AI to adjust light therapy or smart-home environments in real time based on a person's sleep patterns. Newer medications target more specific aspects of sleep regulation, potentially offering treatment options with fewer side effects than some older medications.

Sleep medicine increasingly connects with other medical fields. There is growing recognition that sleep disorders can affect cardiovascular health, mental health conditions, and metabolic processes. This integration across medical specialties reflects a broader understanding that sleep affects many aspects of health rather than being a separate consideration. This collaborative approach may lead to more comprehensive treatment that considers sleep as an important factor in overall health management.

The journey of fully understanding sleep is far from over. My deepest hope is that this book has illuminated the critical importance of sleep and empowered you to optimize your own rest. Sleep is not just a passive state, but an active, transformative experience that touches every aspect of our health, creativity, and potential. If you've gained even a small insight that helps you improve your sleep, then this journey has been worthwhile. Should you wish to share your thoughts, experiences, or questions, I welcome your connection and continued exploration of sleep science. The path to better sleep begins with understanding—and that journey never truly ends.

Index

A
Accelerometer, 29
Accidents, 114
Acetylcholine, 35, 44
Action potential, 4
Adaptive servo-ventilation (ASV), 132
Adenosine, 33, 34, 51
Adenosine triphosphate (ATP), 33
Advanced sleep phase disorder (ASPD), 142
Aging, 153
Alcohol, 54, 127
Alzheimer's disease, 12, 42, 61, 91
Amygdala, 71, 74, 80
Anesthesia, 47
Antibodies, 83, 84
Antidepressants, 74, 120
Antipsychotics, 75, 76
Anxiety, 35, 71, 74, 107, 120
Apnea-Hypopnea Index (AHI), 130
Appetite regulation, 87
Artificial intelligence, 30, 153, 154
Ascending reticular activating system (ARAS), 7, 34, 35
Ashwagandha, 56
Athletes
  poor sleep effects on performance and injury recovery, 107
  poor sleep quality, 107
  sleep optimization, 109
  sleep-deprived, 107, 109
Athletic performance, 107, 109
Augmentation, 139
Automatic positive airway pressure (APAP), 131
Autonomic nervous system, 6
Axon, 4

B
Bedroom temperature, 149
Benzodiazepines, 72, 123, 139
Bi-level positive airway pressure (BiPAP), 132
Bilevel therapy (BiPAP), 129
Biological clocks, 7, 18, 19, 21
Bipolar disorder, 71, 75
Blood-brain barrier, 92
Body mass index (BMI), 126
Blood pressure, 89
Blood sugar, 87
Blood tests, 142
Body temperature, 7, 12, 17, 36, 37, 153
Brain, 3
  activity, 9, 12
  areas in sleep regulation, 34
  brainstem, 3
  glial cells, 3
  neurons, 3
  at night, 33, 35, 36
  structure, 4
  transition from wake to sleep, 33, 35
  wake-promoting system, 33
  waves, 11
Brain activity, 9, 12
Brain imaging studies, 79
Brain imaging techniques, 9
Brainstem, 3
Brain waste clearance pathway, 92
Breast cancer, 95
Breathing disorder, 125, 126
Bruxism, 146
B vitamins, 53

A. Juginovic, *Sleep Science Made Simple*,
https://doi.org/10.1007/978-3-031-92060-8

C

Caffeine, 35, 68, 120, 150
  impact on sleep architecture, 52
  primary action, 51
  and sleep-wake cycle, 51, 52
Carbohydrates, 53
Cardiovascular disease, 89
Cardiovascular health, sleep and, 89
Cardiovascular risk, 133
Cardiovascular system, 89, 133
Central nervous system, 6
Central sleep apnea (CSA), 125, 128
  with Cheyne-Stokes respiration, 128
Cerebrospinal fluid, 12, 42
Chamomile, 56
Chronic insomnia, 55
Chronobiology, 18
Chronotherapy, 23, 122, 144
Chronotypes, 18, 108, 118
Circadian clock, 18
  modern life and, 21–23
Circadian pacemaker, 142
Circadian rhythms, 15, 16, 18, 19, 21–24, 34, 71, 87, 117, 118, 122, 141, 149, 150, 154
  and insomnia risks, 120
  disorders, 23, 141, 142
    diagnosis and treatment, 142, 143
  evolutionary conservation of, 18
  free-running, 21
  impact of, 17
  molecular regulation of, 17
Circulating tumor cells (CTCs), 96
Clonazepam, 139
Clozapine, 76
Coffee nap, 150
Cognitive behavioral therapy for insomnia (CBT-I), 72, 74, 81, 122, 123
Cognitive function, 65, 67, 68, 104
Cognitive impairments, 102
Colorectal cancer, 95
Combined insomnia, 123
Complex sleep apnea syndrome (CompSAS), 125, 129
Congenital paralysis, 46
Consumer Sleep Tech, 29, 30
Continuous positive airway pressure (CPAP) therapy, 129, 131
Cortisol, 5, 79
C-reactive protein, 84
Crohn's disease, 84
CYP1A2 gene, 51
Cytokine, 83

D

Decision-making, 101, 102
Deep sleep, 12, 38, 39, 41–43, 47, 83
Delayed sleep phase disorder (DSPD), 23, 142
Delta waves, 12
Depression, 73, 120
Dim light melatonin onset (DLMO), 117
Dopamine, 35, 137–139
Doxepin, 123
Dreams and brain activity, 45, 46
Drowsy driving, 114

E

Economic impact, 102, 103
Electroencephalography (EEG), 11, 27, 39, 66
Emotional regulation, 81
Estrogen, 52
Eszopiclone, 123
Executive function, 67
Exercise, 150

F

Fatal familial insomnia, 99
Fatigue, 103–105, 113, 114
First Night effect, 28
"Fight or flight" response, 6, 89
Forward-thinking organizations, 104
4-7-8 breathing technique, 122
Functional magnetic resonance imaging (fMRI), 9, 79

G

GABA (gamma-aminobutyric acid), 5, 47, 123
Gabapentin, 139
Gastroesophageal reflux disease (GERD), 84
Genetics, 51, 117, 118, 138, 141
Ghrelin, 87
Glia, 3
Global business operations, 104
GLP-1 receptor agonists, 132
Glycemic index, 53
Glymphatic system, 12, 42, 61, 91
Growth hormone, 12, 42, 92
Gut microbiome, 84

H

Half-life, 51
Hallucination, 76, 147

Health, 153, 154
maintenance, 62
risks, 99, 100
Heart attack, 90, 133
Healthcare, 88
Heart health, 89
Heat transfer, 36
Herbal supplements, 56
High altitude, 128
Hippocampus, 9
Histamine, 35
Hormones, 5
Hypersomnia, 75
Hypnogram, 28
Hypopnea, 125
Hypothalamic-pituitary-adrenal (HPA) axis, 79
Hypothyroidism, 100

I
Immune function, 83
Immune system, 10, 83, 95
Infection susceptibility, 83, 84
Inflammation, 84, 90
Injury prevention, 107
Insomnia, 75, 113, 117, 119
acute, 120
causes of, 120
chronic, 120
diagnosis, 121–124
duration of, 120
episodic, 120
experience of, 119
primary, 120
recovery from chronic, 123
secondary, 120
treatment, 121–124
Insulin, 53, 134
resistance, 87
sensitivity, 124
Interleukin-1, 83
Interleukin-6, 83, 84
Intrinsically photosensitive retinal ganglion cells (ipRGCs), 16, 19, 22
Iron deficiency, 138
anemia, 100
Irregular sleep-wake rhythm disorder, 142

J
Jet lag effect, 109

L
Leadership, 101–103, 105
LED lights, 22
Leptin, 87
Light, 19, 21
Light exposure, 16, 20–23, 150
Light-sensing system, 20
Light sleep, 11, 40
Light therapy, 118, 143
Long-term memory, 65
Loss of consciousness, 46
Lucid dreams, 46

M
Machine learning, 153
Magnesium, 53, 55
Meditation, 40
Melanopsin, 19, 20
Melatonin, 5, 17, 20, 22, 34, 35, 53, 55, 68, 95, 107, 118, 143, 149, 150
Melatonin-rich foods, 54
Memory consolidation, 61
Memory formation, 65
Memory system, 65
Mental health, 71, 72, 114, 121, 134
and sleep disorders, 114
Mental performance, 68
Metabolism, 87
Micro-sleeps, 133
Mindful eating patterns, 11
Mindfulness, 81
meditation, 122
Mindfulness-based stress reduction programs, 81
Motor memory consolidation, 66
Muscle atonia, 12
Muscle relaxation, 122, 151

N
Napping, 150
Nappuccino, 150
Natural killer cells, 81, 83
Neural mechanisms, 67
Neurons, 3, 4
Neurotransmitters, 4, 35, 74
functions, 5
Non-benzodiazepine receptor agonists, 123
"Non-dippers", 89
Non-REM sleep, 11

Non-24-hour sleep-wake disorder, 142
Noradrenaline, 36
Norepinephrine, 35
Normal sleep, 87
Nutrition, 150
  sleep and, 51–55

O
Obesity, 87, 88
Obesity hypoventilation syndrome (OHS), 127
Obstructive sleep apnea (OSA), 125, 127, 132
Olanzapine, 76
Optic nerves, 15, 19
Orexin receptor antagonists, 123
OSA, *see* Obstructive sleep apnea
Oversleeping, 100
Oxidative stress, 92

P
Parasomnias, 43, 145
  in children, 147
  diagnosis, 147
  non REM-related, 146
  prevalence of, 145
  REM-related, 145, 146
  timing of, 145
  treatment, 147
Parasympathetic nervous system, 6, 39, 89, 122
Parkinson's disease, 91, 128, 146
Periodic limb movement disorder (PLMD), 137–139
Peripheral nervous system, 6
Personalized sleep medicine, 117
Pharmacogenomics, 107, 117
Photoreceptors, 19
Physical activity, 11, 37
Pickwickian syndrome, *see* Obesity hypoventilation syndrome (OHS)
Pittsburgh Sleep Quality Index (PSQI), 130
Polygraphy, 28
Polysomnography, 27, 30, 72, 122, 130
Pons, 44
Poor sleep
  athletic performance and injury recovery, effects on, 107, 108
  financial impact of, 102
  leadership skills, effects on, 101, 102
Practical sleep strategies, 151, 152
Pramipexole, 139
Prefrontal cortex, 9, 46, 67
Pregabalin, 139
Process C, 34
Process S, 33
Protein, 16, 53
Pupil, 19

R
Ramelteon, 123
Rapid eye movement (REM) sleep, 10–12, 43, 44, 73, 81
Reactive oxygen species (ROS), 99
Rebound effect, 54
Recovery, 107, 108
Relaxation techniques, 147, 151
REM, *see* Rapid eye movement
REM sleep behavior disorder (RBD), 91, 146
Renin-angiotensin-aldosterone system (RAAS), 89
Respiratory disturbance index (RDI), 130
Restless legs syndrome (RLS), 137–139
Retina, 19
Retinohypothalamic tract, 15, 19
RLS, *see* Restless legs syndrome
Ropinirole, 139

S
Schizophrenia, 71, 75
SCN, *see* Suprachiasmatic nucleus
Selective serotonin reuptake inhibitors (SSRIs), 72, 73
Sensory memory, 65
Serotonin, 53
Serotonin-norepinephrine reuptake inhibitors (SNRIs), 73
Shift work, 95
Sleep, 9, 79, 83, 87, 89, 91, 95, 101
  advances in monitoring technology, 28
  alcohol and, 54
  vs. anesthesia, 46, 47
  and anxiety, 74
  architecture, 11
  and athletes, 107, 109
  balancing, 99
  bedroom temperature for, 11
  bipolar disorder, 75
  brain activity during, 9

and brain health, 91
and cancer risk, 95
and cardiovascular health, 89, 90
changes with age, 10
and depression, 73
in DNA repair, 96
health optimization, role in, 61
hormonal regulation during, 12
hygiene, 11
and immune function, 83
impacts on metabolic health, 87
and injury rehabilitation, 108
interventions, 76
in learning and cognitive effects of poor sleep, 65–69
and mental health, 71, 72
nutrition and, 51–54, 56
poor sleep effects on leadership skills, 101, 102
quality, 62, 75, 80, 84, 108
regulation, 34
REM, 43, 44
and schizophrenia, 75, 76
shift work and, 95
spindles, 41, 66
stage distribution through night, 29
stage N1 (light and short), 39, 40
stage N2, 40, 41
stage N3 (deep sleep), 42
stages, 9, 38–44
and stress, 79, 81
study, 27, 28, 30
supplements, 55, 56
and temperature, 36, 37
Sleep apnea, 92, 93, 113, 114, 122, 125
alcohol consumption and, 127
central sleep apnea (CSA), 128
with Cheyne-Stokes respiration, 128
complex sleep apnea syndrome (CompSAS), 129
diagnosis and treatment, 130–132
gender influences, 126
lifestyle factors, 127
obstructive sleep apnea (OSA), 127
risk factors and prevalence, 126
types of, 127–129
untreated, long-term impact of, 133, 134
Sleep apps, 30
Sleep architecture, 11
caffeine impact, 52
Sleep deprivation, 61, 65–67, 74, 88, 99, 103, 120
Sleep disorders, 81, 113, 117, 119, 137, 149, 152–154
mental health and, 114
physical health impact of, 113
workplace impact of, 114
Sleep disruption, 71–73, 75, 83, 84, 114
Sleep disturbances, 72, 73
Sleep duration, 100
Sleep-friendly practices, 104
Sleep hormone, *see* Melatonin
Sleep hygiene, 11, 105, 122
Sleep loss, 74, 99
Sleep medicine, 113, 117, 118
future of, 153, 154
Sleep monitoring, 28
Sleep-onset insomnia, 123
Sleep optimization
daily habits and sleep, 150
environmental factors, 149
exercise, 150
light exposure, 150
nutrition and sleep, 150
practical sleep strategies, 151, 152
strategic napping, 150
time and consistency, 149
Sleep paralysis, 147
Sleep patterns, 11, 12
Sleep pressure, 5, 34
Sleep quality, 11, 150–152
Sleep regulation, 5
Sleep-related eating disorder, 146
Sleep restoration, 61
Sleep restriction, 122
therapy, 81
Sleep science, future of, 153, 154
Sleep stages, 9, 37–45
Sleep state misperception, 122
Sleep terrors, 145, 146
Sleep timing, 16, 17, 21
Sleep tracking, 27, 30
Sleep-wake cycle, 141, 142
Sleep-wake regulation, neural circuit, 16
Sleepwalking, 146, 147
Slow-wave sleep, 66
Smart mattresses, 30
Social jet lag, 18, 23
Somnambulism, 146
Spinal cord, 3
Stimulus control, 81
STOP-Bang questionnaire, 130
Strategic napping, 150
Stress, 35, 79, 119, 120
Stress hormone, *see* Cortisol
Stress management, 147
Stroke, 90, 128, 133
Supplements, sleep, 55, 56

Suprachiasmatic nucleus (SCN), 4, 15, 19, 141, 143, 149
Suvorexant, 123
Sympathetic nervous system, 7, 9

T
Technology, 154
Teeth grinding, 146
Temazepam, 123
Temperature regulation, 7
Temperature sensitivity, 37
T helper cells, 84
Theta waves, 11
Thyroid stimulating hormone (TSH), 5
Time givers, 21
T lymphocytes, 83
Training optimization, 108, 109
Treatment, 113, 114
Triazolam, 123
Tryptophan, 53
Tryptophan-rich foods, 54, 150
Tumor necrosis factor-alpha, 83
Type 2 diabetes, 87, 134

U
Ulcerative colitis, 84
Uvulopalatopharyngoplasty, 132

V
Valerian root, 56
Vasopressin, 55
Ventrolateral preoptic nucleus (VLPO), 34
Virtual meetings, 103

W
Wearable devices, 29
Workplace, 103–105, 114
  culture, 102, 104
  safety, 114
World Health Organization, 73

Z
Zaleplon, 123
Z-drugs, 123
Zolpidem, 123

MIX
Papier aus verantwortungsvollen Quellen
Paper from responsible sources
FSC® C105338

If you have any concerns about our products,
you can contact us on
ProductSafety@springernature.com

In case Publisher is established outside the EU,
the EU authorized representative is:
Springer Nature Customer Service Center GmbH
Europaplatz 3, 69115 Heidelberg, Germany

Printed by Libri Plureos GmbH
in Hamburg, Germany